Enhancing Wellness

CAROLYN CHAMBERS CLARK, R.N., Ed.D., F.A.A.N., is Director of The Wellness Institute (an organization devoted to providing consultation, educational experiences, and research on wellness topics), and Editor of the *Wellness Newsletter.*

Enhancing Wellness

A GUIDE FOR SELF-CARE

Carolyn Chambers Clark, R.N., Ed.D., F.A.A.N.

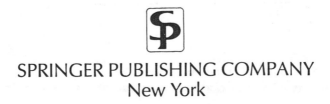

SPRINGER PUBLISHING COMPANY
New York

The material presented for enhancing wellness has been carefully researched and tried out for accuracy and safety. The
author and publisher, however, disclaim any responsibility for
any adverse effects or consequences resulting from the misap-
plication or injudicious use of any of the material presented in
this book.

Springer Publishing Company, Inc.
200 Park Avenue South
New York, N.Y. 10003

82 83 84 85 / 10 9 8 7 6 5 4 3 2

Library of Congress Cataloging in Publication Data

Clark, Carolyn Chambers.
    Enhancing Wellness.

        Bibliography: p.
        Includes index.
        1. Health.   2. Health behavior.   3. Self-care,
Health.   I. Title.   [DNLM: 1. Health.   QT 255 C592e]
RA776.C5467   613   80-26994
ISBN 0-8261-2950-1
ISBN 0-8261-2951-X (pbk.)

Printed in the United States of America

For my mother, Phyllis O. Stark,
who started me on my journey toward wellness

CONTENTS

PREFACE

Enhancing Wellness provides information pertaining to wellness and health promotion. Assessment guides and practice exercises appear as figures throughout the book. These will help you to assess various aspects of wellness and take action to enhance your wellness, should you choose to do so.

The book is devoted to six dimensions of wellness. The dimensions are aspects of wellness that interact with and affect one another. A high level of wellness is a dynamically balanced one, where nutrition, self-healing, exercise, environmental sensitivity, caring, stress, self-responsibility, and self-care are blended. Since no one dimension can lead to wellness, chapter divisions are somewhat arbitrary and limiting. It is hoped you will bear with this limitation and remember that each dimension affects and is affected by every other.

A major theme throughout the book is that your level of wellness rests to a large degree on your actions and not on the actions of others. Many of the suggested methods work very well in combination with more traditional health care practices. *Enhancing Wellness* is not meant to replace the relationship you have with a physician or other health care practitioner. In fact, part of the book is devoted to working more closely with such a person. This book does *not* take the stand that you should attempt to care for yourself without the support of more traditional care when you are in a critical or emergency situation or when you have a diagnosed illness. Many of the materials provided in the practice exercises can, however, be used in combination with more conventional medical practices even under emergency and illness conditions. And, if you take the suggested actions presented herein, you will be less likely to incur some of the more common chronic illnesses and will probably find yourself relying less and less on a physician or other health care practitioner. This book *is* meant to empower you to take action toward wellness. The initial steps are the most difficult and anxiety-provoking. Writing this book has forced me to examine my life style and to change those parts that decrease my level of wellness. It has not been an easy road, and although I feel more energetic and alive, I have also realized that a wellness approach demands constant attention and work. For those who feel up to the task and the benefits to be derived—read on.

Best wishes on your journey,

Carolyn Chambers Clark

acknowledgments

I want to thank Dr. John Diamond and Harper & Row for permission to quote parts of the muscle test from *Behavioral Kinesiology*; Gloria Serra for her industrious typing of the manuscript; and Sue DiFabio and Judith Ackerhalt for their critical support during the planning stages of the book.

C. C. C.

Enhancing Wellness

1

Health and Wellness

Many people are puzzled by the word, *wellness*. Health, on the other hand, has so many connotations that people are not clear on the meaning of that term either. Defining health in terms of statistics such as numbers of deaths or incidences of illness continues to be a common practice [1]. Yet, the Constitution of the World Health Organization declares that health is not simply the absence of disease or infirmity [2]. This chapter explores the meanings of health and wellness and provides a basic wellness self-assessment.

HEALTH IS RELATED TO LIFE STYLE

Once it is agreed that individuals are responsible for their health because they are responsible for their life style, there will be less need to place the burden for all that happens or does not happen in the health field on physicians. By clarifying the definition of health and medical care, it will be possible for us to see more clearly who is responsible [3]. Health care and medical care are often considered synonymous by caregivers and clients; in fact, medical care is only one part of health care. Another part of health care is self-care, or the process of functioning on one's own behalf to promote health and to detect and prevent illness [4].

It is a fact that health is related to life style and environmental factors. This fact is being backed up daily by research that has shown that the risk of becoming ill can be predicted by the number and type of life changes a person is subjected to [5]. Smoking has been linked to cancer of the lung, larynx, lip, oral cavity, esophagus, bladder and other urinary organs, chronic bronchitis and emphysema, arteriosclerotic heart disease, a shorter life, and to the physical problems of children born of smoking mothers. Alcohol is a factor in half of all motor vehicle fatalities, half of all homicides, and one-third of all suicides and results in a loss of $15 billion in work productivity, cirrhosis of the liver, malnutrition, lowered resistance to infectious diseases, gastrointestinal irritations, muscle diseases and tremors, brain and nervous system damage, and physical problems in children born of mothers who drink [6]. Five of the ten leading causes of death—heart and cerebrovascular diseases, diabetes mellitus, arteriosclerosis, and cirrhosis of the liver—are diet-related [7]. Coffee, tea, cola drinks, and other substances containing caffeine are suspect because caffeine induces stomach acid secretion leading to heartburn, bleeding ulcers, and nervousness due to B-vitamin excretion [8]. Chronic stress can lead to migraine headaches, peptic ulcers, heart attacks, hypertension, mental illness, suicide, strokes, bowel disorders, diabetes mellitus, and some skin disorders [9, 10]. Inactivity or lack of exercise has convincingly been linked to hypertension, chronic fatigue, physiological inefficiency, premature aging, poor musculature, and inadequate flexibility. These conditions then contribute to lower-back pain, injury, tension, obesity, and coronary heart disease [11, 12]. Overnutrition contributes to 50 percent of all cancers [13]. Hope and faith correlate with healing, and depression and feelings of chronic anxiety and hostility are correlated with cancer [14]. Among the underlying causes of elevated blood pressure are emotional stress, obesity, dietary salt, and smoking [15].

Although these facts are frightening, they are also enlightening, for they show how much individuals can control their health. They can take responsibility for what is eaten, drunk, and smoked and obtain appropriate exercise, reduce stress, and use self-healing measures.

A *holistic* view of health takes into account every possible concept and skill that could enhance wellness. It is a view that attempts to help the person to grow toward harmony and balance, whereby the person is helped, rather than a disease treated. Natural methods are used when possible, but the best of modern Western medicine is used, too. In a holistic approach, the person engages in a healthier style of living. The interrelationships between body, mind, and spirit are promoted and enhanced. In this view, body symptoms or psychic pain are viewed as messages we give ourselves to eat less or differently, to exercise more, to reduce stress, to grieve when grief is called for, to rearrange our work or living environment, or to increase responsibility or concern. Thus, illness is seen as a message from within—the meaning of which can be defined and from which growth can occur. Wellness depends on taking assertive action and on having a broad view of different conditions or situations that precede problems, not only on dealing with symptoms of distress. Waiting for a headache or a cold or cancer or high blood pressure to occur leaves people at a disadvantage, because they must wait passively to see whether they will be healthy or not. Wellness requires confidence in the future. Those who have—or aspire to have—high-level wellness make decisions about their own health; they participate in it and create it, and they know how to assess an imbalance *before* chronic illness strikes. They know the factors that create imbalance, such as eating highly refined, processed foods, wearing clothes made of synthetic fibers, being exposed to poisons and noise from the environment, having poor posture and constant muscle tension, or being exposed to constant stressful relationships at school, work, or home without using stress-reduction techniques. People interested in holistic health promote it through education in the components of well-being and their interaction [16].

YOU AS CLIENT

This is where you come in—as your own *client* in holistic health action, and possibly as role model and facilitator of others' health. The word, "client," implies that the person seeking help takes some responsibility for the relationship or for how things proceed. In other words, the client is not a passive recipient of knowledge or of directives, but an active participant. The idea that people can participate in their own health and care is not new; in fact, studies show that at least 75 percent of all health care is self-provided. Most of the problems diagnosed by physicians are self-limiting without any treatment [17], and many physical complaints brought to doctors are pleas for sympathy, reassurance, and encouragement [18]. Besides, our bodies have intuitive knowledge of how to heal themselves, provided we do not get in the way; in blood cells, substances from the external environment are analyzed and antibodies are developed to neutralize harmful ones [19]. Hope and faith are other tools everyone has to facilitate healing. In fact, when these tools are lacking, people may not heal, they may develop cancer or other illnesses, or they may die prematurely [20]. When physicians diagnose terminal illnesses and their clients recover, doctors often call it a spontaneous remission. Other physicians call it the will to live or the will to be healed [21].

One way you can begin to have a more active role in your own wellness is through using a wellness contract. You can make this contract with yourself or with your health care practitioner or health educator. Figure 1–1 gives an example of a contract made by one woman with herself.

DIMENSIONS OF WELLNESS

One way to view the dimensions of wellness is to consider physical, psychological, and social aspects. The physical aspect is the easiest to define, as it includes everything taken into the body, such as food, water, and air. It also includes everything put out of the body, such as energy for exercise, eliminating waste, and healing. It further includes reducing stress through activities such as warm baths, massage, or relaxation exercises.

The psychological dimension is harder to define. Just as there is a muscle tightness derived from incorrect or insufficient physical output, in the same way there is a tightness derived from an inner attitude of self-dislike [22]. People who judge themselves severely expend a great deal of energy keeping emotionally tight and locked up. They set unrealistically high standards for themselves and punish themselves when they do not attain these unattainable goals. Those who have attained a high level of wellness like themselves and their accomplishments, and they are not totally dependent on others for their own well-being. Attaining a high level of wellness in the psychological aspect also means realizing that each of us is responsible for our own feelings, that we can no longer blame others if we feel hurt, angry, or sad. Another part of psychological wellness is the ability to *really* listen to ourselves and others, to be empathic by understanding the words and the feeling or intent behind the words.

Although physical and psychological aspects have been presented as if they are separate, they really interact with one another and with social and spiritual aspects. For example, if people live in a tense situation, dislike their work, or have an imbalance between intensity and relaxation, they are bound to feel poorly physically and mentally.

The interrelatedness of the various aspects has been explained in the following way:

> Therefore what on the physical plane is illness, on the psychological plane depression or anxiety, is on the spiritual plane alienation: The feeling of being cut off, separate, uninvolved, isolated [23].

This interrelatedness is also visible in those who begin to eat better or to exercise more. They often report an increase in the number of spiritual experiences called oneness, peak experience, or enlightenment. This need to feel a part of something greater than oneself is the spiritual side of us. People cannot attain a high level of wellness if they are constantly defending themselves against a hostile environment [24]. Healthy people do not disregard danger, but they are not constantly under threat from "something out there."

Another way to view wellness is to define specific activities that tend to lead to wellness. Again, although the various activities will be discussed separately, there is a great deal of interaction between them. At the end of this chapter there is a wellness assessment called, "How Well Am I?" This assessment is divided into sections: *Eating well, Being fit, Feeling good, Caring for self/others, Fitting in*, and *Being responsible*. There is much overlap and many of the questions relate to more than one of the activities; but then, that is how it should be in a holistic approach to wellness.

Eating well encompasses everything that is taken into the body; it also entails digestion and elimination. If you eat the right food but are unable to absorb nutrients, suffer from indigestion or gas, or are unable to eliminate waste, your nutritional needs will not have been met. Eating well means maximizing the use of fresh, uncooked fruits and vegetables and whole grains, and minimizing the use of saturated fats, coffee, tea, cola drinks, alcohol, and highly processed foods that contain harmful additives, flavors, or colorings. The first section of the assessment, "How Well Am I?" will help you to assess this dimension.

Being fit encompasses exercise, flexibility, circulation, and general body fitness including the ability to heal and to recover from illness. You will notice that there are some statements in this section that overlap with other sections. In fact, the statements are divided into dimensions only to increase your ease of taking or administering the assessment. You will notice in this section as well as in others that your own satisfaction with your nutrition, fitness, and so on is considered as important as more "objective" measures of wellness.

Feeling good encompasses ability to reduce stress, to rest, relax, and employ a sense of humor. Spreading out life changes, sleeping well, saying no to others' requests, the ability to use relaxation techniques and/or creative visualization, and successful grieving of losses or separations are examples of ways of reducing stress and feeling good. In this dimension—as in the others—there is an underlying idea that it is balance that is healthy; for example, it is important to be able to balance seriousness with humor, and exercise that conditions the heart with exercise that increases body flexibility and relaxation.

Caring for includes both taking care of oneself and caring for others; again, balance in these two leads to wellness. Too much of one or the other decreases level of wellness. Caring, healing, using healthy ways to care for self, having a sense of purpose and optimism, speaking up for rights in an assertive way, empathy, and sharing with others are all intimately connected and related. Caring for includes a sense of belonging to groups and the larger community and liking oneself sufficiently.

Fitting in encompasses unity or fit with the physical and social environment. There is a strong sense of conserving the earth's resources rather than wasting them. It includes learning to design and shape the home, work, and social environments that are under the client's control.

Being responsible encompasses taking responsibility for one's own health, taking safe action toward wellness, clarifying values about wellness and acting on them, and generally acting as a responsible citizen. Being responsible also includes making well-thought-out decisions, not impulsive, unthinking ones. The dimension of being responsible overrides and interacts with all other dimensions and is a major factor in balancing aspects of other dimensions, for example being sure you take care of yourself as well as others. Although this book goes into detail about how to enhance wellness, there are a few things that anyone can do to increase life expectancy, such as [25]:

have breakfast every day

eat three meals a day

avoid snacks

have moderate exercise two or three times a week

get seven to eight hours sleep every night

do not smoke

ingest no alcohol or only drink in moderation

keep weight moderate

The remaining chapters in this book will help you to examine and help to change patterns of eating, staying fit, feeling good, caring, and being responsible. The Appendix provides a wealth of information about wellness resources. Figure 1–2 can be used to help you assess your degree of wellness.

Figure 1–1 Sample Contract

---

1. The major ways I want to live more healthfully are:

    a. to jog daily

    b. to cut down on desserts except fresh fruit

    c. to practice relaxation exercises daily to reduce stress

    d. to anticipate changes and spread them out if I can

2. Specific actions I plan to take to become more healthy are:

    a. jog in the morning when I have the most energy

    b. not buy any sweets except fresh fruit

    c. set aside ten minutes before bedtime for relaxing

    d. make a list of known upcoming changes

3. Since I know myself, I know I might try to sabotage my efforts by:

    a. telling myself I'm too busy to jog

    b. feeling tired right before jogging

    c. "forgetting" to jog

    d. rationalizing desserts by saying I need to reward myself

4. I will know when I have met my contract when:

    a. I have jogged daily for six months

    b. I no longer crave sweets

    c. I am able to relax my body at will—at work or at home

    d. I face no more than two planned changes at any one time

---

Figure 1-2 /// 9

Figure 1-2   How Well Am I?

Directions:

Try to respond to the statements that follow in a yes/no fashion. The statements are divided into six categories, but you will notice that many could be placed in more than one category; this is not unusual in a holistic approach where the whole person is being focused on. When you have answered all six parts, complete the questions that follow.

EATING WELL   Yes   No

1.   I maximize fresh fruits and uncooked vegetables in my diet   ....

2.   I minimize the use of candy, sweets, and sugar   ....

3.   I eat whole-grain breads and cereals   ....

4.   I avoid foods that have color, artificial flavor, or preservatives added to them   ....

5.   I eat unsaturated fats, such as cold pressed vegetable oils, lean meat, fish, and chicken   ....

6.   I avoid meats that contain drugs or feed additives (beef, chicken, pork)   ....

7.   I avoid coffee, tea, cola drinks, or other substances that are high in caffeine or stimulants   ....

8.   I eat foods that are high in roughage, or I try to take bran daily   ....

9.   I read labels on packaged goods and stay away from highly processed foods   ....

10. I have a good appetite, but I eat sensible amounts of food   ....

11. I eat only when I am hungry   ....

12. I eat only when I feel relaxed   ....

13. I am satisfied with what I eat   ....

14. I drink enough water so my urine is light yellow   ....

15. I know the foods and drugs I am allergic to, and I never take them   ....

16. I avoid drinking alcohol in any form   ....

17. I avoid fatty foods (beef, lamb, pork, soft cheeses, gravies, ice cream, fried foods, etc.)   ....

(continued)

Figure 1-2   (continued)

	Yes	No
18. I avoid all "junk" foods, such as hot dogs, potato chips, sugary breakfast cereals, etc.	......	......
19. I avoid all food or food products that have been suspected of increasing potential for cancer, such as saccharin, Red No. 40, synthetic coal tar dyes, foods labeled FD and C or U.S. Certified color, bacon, sandwich meats, salami, bologna, smoked meats and fish, any food containing torula yeast, or organ meats (liver, pancreas, sweetbreads, or kidney)	......	......
20. I have installed and use an activated carbon filtration system to my drinking water tap to remove organic contaminants	......	......

BEING FIT

	Yes	No
1. I weigh within ten percent of my desirable weight	......	......
2. I feel my body is under my control	......	......
3. I walk up one flight of stairs rather than take an elevator or escalator, and I walk rather than travel by car when possible	......	......
4. I walk an hour, jog, or exercise vigorously at least three times a week	......	......
5. My muscles are firm and well-developed	......	......
6. I do flexibility or stretching exercises daily	......	......
7. I have a good sense of balance and walk confidently	......	......
8. My joints are flexible and free from pain	......	......
9. My eyes are clear, and my vision is adequate	......	......
10. My hearing is good	......	......
11. My nose and sinuses feel O.K. and work well	......	......
12. My tongue and gums are pink	......	......
13. My mouth and throat feel O.K. and work well	......	......
14. My neck feels and looks O.K.	......	......
15. My skin, hair, and fingernails are in good condition	......	......

Figure 1-2 /// 11

	Yes	No
16. I breathe easily and well	......	......
17. I seem to digest my food well	......	......
18. I have at least one well-formed, large bowel movement a day with ease and comfort	......	......
19. I am satisfied with my sexual activities	......	......
20. I rarely get injuries	......	......
21. I am satisfied with my body condition	......	......
22. My pulse is 70 beats per minute or less	......	......
23. When I look at my body, it looks healthy and strong	......	......
24. When I do get sick, I'm resilient and I recover pretty easily	......	......

For premenopausal women

25. I have a regular menstrual period with little discomfort	......	......

FEELING GOOD

1. I sleep well	......	......
2. I have a peaceful expectation about death	......	......
3. I live relatively free from pain and limiting illness	......	......
4. I live relatively free from disabling stress or painful, repetitive thoughts	......	......
5. I can laugh at myself occasionally, and I have a good sense of humor	......	......
6. I have discovered safe ways of releasing my frustration and anger	......	......
7. I try to spread out predictable events and changes in my life to keep them from happening at once	......	......
8. I try to stay away from overly noisy, crowded, smoky, or unsafe places	......	......
9. I respect my accomplishments	......	......
10. When people trample on my rights, I speak up for myself in an assertive way	......	......

(continued)

Figure 1-2 (continued)

		Yes	No
11.	I allow myself to rest, to be quiet, and/or to meditate occasionally	....	....
12.	I can say no to others' requests without feeling guilty	....	....
13.	I am satisfied with my ability to relax	....	....
14.	If I close my eyes, I can visualize myself in a quiet, peaceful, restful scene, *or* I can relax parts of my body if I concentrate on doing so	....	....
15.	I know most of the changes that are affecting me today	....	....
16.	I feel accepting of and calm about people or things I have lost through separation or death	....	....
17.	I feel good about my relationships with younger people or children	....	....
18.	I feel good about my relationships with older people or parents	....	....
19.	I am aware of my feelings and express them to others in a way that is satisfying to me	....	....
20.	I am able to cope with a reasonable amount of stress	....	....
21.	I use my sense of creativity and play	....	....
22.	Depending on the situation, I can move easily from seriousness to easy, good humor	....	....
23.	I am satisfied with the amount of touching and hugging I give to and get from others	....	....
24.	I look forward to each new day	....	....
25.	I feel good about myself	....	....

CARING FOR SELF/OTHERS

1.	I practice self-healing measures	....	....
2.	I live with a sense of concern for others	....	....
3.	I think my attitude and my general health are important to how well I heal	....	....

Figure 1-2 /// 13

		Yes	No

4. I have at least one other person with whom I can discuss my innermost thoughts and feelings ....

5. I like being alone as well as being with others ....

6. When I get a headache or feel pain, I try other comfort measures before I reach for aspirin or other drugs ....

7. When I get tense or nervous, I try other measures before I reach for drugs or alcohol ....

8. I avoid smoking, and I try to avoid those who smoke ....

9. I watch out for myself so I am hardly ever involved in "accidents" ....

10. When others need or ask for help from me, I am able to respond in a helpful way ....

11. I try to keep myself open to new experiences ....

12. I have good listening skills, and I listen to others' words *and* the feelings behind the words ....

FITTING IN

1. I feel as if I fit in my spot in the universe ....

2. I can work well with different groups of people ....

3. My friends practice a wellness life style ....

4. I have designed my personal environment (living quarters, workplace) to suit me ....

Conserving the earth's resources

5. I live in a well-insulated home ....

6. I turn lights off when I am not using them ....

7. I buy and use as few electrical appliances and gadgets as possible ....

8. I grow at least some of the food I eat ....

9. I eat foods that require less energy to produce (rice, beans, wheat, barley, oats) ....

10. I dress warmly rather than turn up the heat ....

(continued)

Figure 1-2 (continued)

		Yes	No
11.	I have fewer children or adopt those already born	......	......
12.	I use trimmings from uncooked fruits and vegetables to fertilize my garden	......	......
13.	I have cut back on using disposable and convenience items	......	......
14.	I buy recycled items when I can	......	......

Protecting myself from dangers in the environment

		Yes	No
15.	When I can I buy fruits that have not been sprayed with dangerous pesticides	......	......
16.	I do not live close to a major highway, *or* I use nutritional, exercise, or self-healing measures to reduce the effects of carbon monoxide and other airborne chemicals	......	......
17.	I work in a place that provides adequate personal space, comfort, safety, direct sunlight, and fresh air from open windows, and where air, water, or material pollutants are limited, *or* I use nutritional, exercise, or stress reduction measures to minimize negative effects	......	......
18.	My home does not have asbestos insulation or asbestos lining of ventilation and heating ducts	......	......
19.	I refrain from using pesticides for termite treatment or other purposes such as gardening; instead, I use biological control through pest management systems	......	......
20.	I avoid using cosmetics carrying the label: "Warning: the safety of this product has not been determined"	......	......
21.	I avoid using permanent hair dyes or cosmetics containing: Yellow No.1, Blue No.6, and Reds Nos.10, 11, 12, and 13 (the red colors used in lipstick and soap)	......	......
22.	I avoid x-rays unless serious disease or injury is at stake, and I have dental x-rays for diagnostic reasons only every three to five years	......	......
23.	I avoid all aerosol sprays	......	......

Figure 1-2 /// 15

	Yes	No

24. I avoid using agents or solvents containing carbon tetrachloride, trichloroethylene, perchloroethylene, or benzene

BEING RESPONSIBLE

1. I persevere to get things I want
2. I know what I value, and I live according to my values
3. I frequently examine my values and actions to see that I am moving toward a wellness orientation
4. My values about health and wellness and the way I act are in accord
5. I live with a sense of purpose to my life
6. I know my pulse, respiration, and blood pressure
7. When I visit a doctor, nurse, lawyer, or other professional person, I ask them how they can help me and how we can work together
8. I am satisfied with the amount of responsibility I take for what happens to me
9. I am able to make decisions in a clear, logical way
10. If a doctor were to tell me I need surgery or that I am to take a medication over a long period of time, I would see at least one other doctor for another opinion
11. I ask others around me not to smoke
12. I vote regularly and keep informed on important issues
13. I avoid drinking when I drive or riding with drivers who drink
14. I wear seat belts when driving, and I insist that those who ride with me do too
15. I know what chronic illnesses my parents and grandparents had, and I take special steps to avoid incurring those illnesses

(continued)

Figure 1–2 (continued)

		Yes	No
16.	I balance my energy between giving to others and getting things I need	......	......
17.	I prepare for upcoming situations by thinking them through and practicing what I will do in the actual situation	......	......
18.	I carry a card with me at all times listing my blood type, food or drug allergies, and chronic illnesses	......	......
19.	I wear a good sunscreen ointment when working or relaxing in the sun	......	......
20.	I look up all medications prescribed for me in an up-to-date reference book, and I carefully read the label and insert in packaged medicines	......	......

For parents with school-age children

21.	I check to make sure that my children go to school in a location far away from chemical, mining, or smelting plants and expressways or highways *or* take steps to protect them from the effects of such situations	......	......
22.	I work to ban the use of junk or convenience foods in cafeterias or schools	......	......
23.	I check to ensure my children are not exposed to harmful chemicals in laboratory courses	......	......
24.	I ensure that my children do not use sleepwear that has been treated with the flame retardant Tris	......	......

For people who work in high-risk industries: petrochemical, asbestos, steel, smelting, and some mining

25.	I work in a job where I am completely informed of the type and effects of the chemicals I use	......	......

For fertile men and women

26.	I take precautions against pregnancy, unless my partner and I have agreed that we want a baby	......	......

Figure 1-2   ///   17

QUESTIONS TO PONDER

1. To how many statements did you answer "no"?

2. Do you think your "nos" are representative of your state of wellness?

3. Do you need more information on why certain statements were included? If so, some of the information appears later in this book, and you may wish to search for it, as well as look up additional material.

4. Are you satisfied with your state of wellness?

5. If you are not satisfied, what specific steps do you plan to take so you will be more satisfied?

NOTES

1. *Conference on Future Directions in Health Care: The Dimensions of Medicine.* Chicago, Blue Cross Association, 1975, p. 98. Proceedings of a conference sponsored on Dec. 10 and 11, 1975, in New York City by Blue Cross, The Rockefeller Foundation, and the Health Policy Program of the University of California School of Medicine, San Francisco.
2. Ibid., pp. 139–141.
3. *Health. United States 1976–1977*, DHEW Publication No. (HRA) 77-1232. Washington, D.C.: U.S. Government Printing Office, 1977, p. 47.
4. Halbert L. Dunn. "High level wellness for man and society," *American Journal of Public Health* 49, no. 6 (1959), p. 786.
5. Thomas H. Holmes. *Schedule of Recent Experience.* Seattle: Department of Psychiatry and Behavioral Sciences, University of Washington School of Medicine. n.d.
6. *Forward Plan for Health: FY 1975–81.* Washington, D.C.: U.S. Department of Health, Education and Welfare, 1975, pp. 100–101.
7. U.S. Senate Select Committee on Nutrition and Human Needs. *Nutrition and Health: An Evaluation of Nutritional Surveillance in the United States.* Washington, D.C.: U.S. Government Printing Office, 1975, p. 5.
8. Donald B. Ardell. *High Level Wellness.* Emmaus, Pa.: Rodale, 1977, p. 119.
9. Hans Selye. *Stress without Distress.* New York: Lippincott, 1974, p. 111.
10. Herbert Benson. *The Relaxation Response.* New York: Avon, 1975, p. 29.
11. *Forward Plan for Health*, p. 108.
12. L. E. Morehouse and Leonard Gross. *Total Fitness in 30 Minutes a Week.* New York: Pocket Books, 1976, p. 21.
13. *Conference on Future Directions in Health Care*, pp. 51-52.
14. Ibid., pp. 63-77.
15. *Forward Plan for Health*, p. 36.
16. Ardell, *High Level Wellness*, p. 47.
17. Sandra Rosenzweig. "Learning to be your own M.D.," *New York Times Magazine*, April 2, 1978, p. 45.
18. Sam M. Cordes. "Assessing health care needs: elements and processes," *Family and Community Health* 1, no. 2 (1978), p. 4.
19. Mike Samuels and Hal Bennett. *The Well Body Book.* New York: Random House, 1973, p. 1.
20. *Conference on Future Directions*, pp. 63-65.
21. Richard Shames and Chuck Sterin. *Healing with Mind Power.* Emmaus, Pa.: Rodale, 1978, p. 5.
22. Ibid., p. 162.
23. Ibid., p. 166.
24. Ibid., pp. 166-167.
25. Donald Vickery. *Life Plan For Your Health*, Reading, Mass.: Addison-Wesley, 1978, p. 23.

2

Eating Well

This chapter focuses on what is taken into the body, used, and eliminated. Some topics that will be surveyed are food myths, suggested dietary goals, vitamins, minerals, cholesterol, fiber, food allergies, the production, purchase, and preparation of food, ingesting chemicals, diet during stress and at special times, digesting well, and personalizing nutrition. It is wise to keep in mind that good nutrition, digestion, and elimination are only parts of a wellness approach; they need to be considered together with ways of reducing stress, of fitting in socially and ecologically, of obtaining appropriate exercise, of caring for self and others, and of having self-responsibility for actions.

Until recently, there has been a strong focus on microbes as the cause of disease; as a result, although there has been research to back the importance of nutrition in the occurrence of disease, few health care practitioners have learned about the preventive aspects of nutrition [1]. In fact, according to a government study, poor nutrition is associated with "six of the ten leading causes of death, including heart disease, some cancers, stroke and hypertension, arteriosclerosis, diabetes, and cirrhosis of the liver"[2]. The study of nutrition should, therefore, be an area of concern for everyone.

FOOD MYTHS

There are several myths about the body's need for protein and how that need can be met. One of these is that meat contains more protein than do other foods. Actually, meat contains only about 25 percent protein, and thus it falls about the middle of the protein quantity scale, ranking below soybeans, fish, milk, soybean flour, and eggs [3]. Another myth is that one must eat a large quantity of meat in order to get sufficient protein to grow and to replace skin, hair, nails, cartilage, tendons, and muscles, to prevent too much base or acid in the blood, to regulate the body's water balance, and to form new antibodies to fight infection. The fact is that Americans eat almost twice the amount of protein their bodies can use; they could get the recommended daily allowances of protein (53 to 58 grams) even if they completely eliminated meat, fish, and poultry from their diet [4]. Another myth is that meat has the highest quality protein available. *Quality* of protein really means how much of the protein that is eaten is actually used by the body. Eggs and milk are more usable by the body than meat is, and soybeans and whole rice are as usable.

Usability relates to amino acids. Our bodies use proteins made up of 22 amino acids; eight of these must be obtained from food, while the others are manufactured in the body. All eight amino acids must be obtained daily and simultaneously, or the manufacture of protein will drop or stop. In addition, these amino acids are essential to life and must be available in a given proportion: for example, peanuts alone do not supply the right pattern or amount of essential amino acids, whereas meat, eggs, and some cheeses alone do. But, by combining wheat and beans, milk and rice, milk and peanuts, or beans and rice, the deficient amino acids in one food are supplemented by the other. Such combinations increase the protein quality *above* the average of the items eaten separately [5]. There are other combinations that can provide adequate protein, but complementing foods takes some skill and know-how and additional knowledge that is beyond the scope of this book. You may wish to refer to Frances Moore Lappe's *Diet for a Small Planet* [3] for further information on the subject.

Another myth about meat is that it is the sole source of some essential vitamins and minerals. In fact, except for Vitamin B_{12}—and this vitamin is found in dairy products—it is nonmeat sources that provide more than half the vitamins and minerals most often cited, and these sources can provide the rest also, often in greater quantities.

For example, baked potatoes and lima beans contain more potassium than does meat, and cocoa, nuts, soybeans, whole grains, and green leafy vegetables contain more magnesium[6].

There is a common myth that "sugar is sugar." But there are naturally occurring sugars in milk, fruits, and vegetables that enhance wellness, whereas table sugar or refined sugar—which is placed in coffee, or found in soft drinks or fancy desserts and many processed foods—is detrimental to health. The primary advantage of using sugars from natural sources is that other nutrients are also available in the food, whereas refined sugar is totally lacking in these nutrients. A label stating that the food within the container is "natural" does not mean that there is no refined sugar in it.

Another myth about sugar is that it is a good source of energy, and people are apt to drink sodas or eat candy bars to "get more energy." Actually, eating refined sugar leads to *less* energy because the food is digested quickly, and the blood level of sugar (glucose) rises very rapidly. As a result, insulin is dumped in excess into the blood and liver reserves of glycogen (stored glucose) are used, and this leads to fatigue, shakiness, irritability, faintness, and, in some cases, violent behavior. It also leads to a harmful cycle of taking in more sugar to "get a lift." For high energy, frequent high-protein meals are recommended. Cravings for sweets will decrease over time. Occasional cravings can be assuaged by eating a piece of fresh or dried fruit.

Another myth is that carbohydrates are "starch" and, if eaten, lead to overweight. But complex carbohydrates such as those contained in fruits, vegetables, and whole-grain cereals and breads do not add weight unless they are combined with fats or with refined sugar. For example, a baked potato stuffed with low-fat cottage cheese is a low-calorie addition to a meal, and one that furnishes many vitamins, minerals, and useful protein. On the other hand, refined sugar and high-fat milk on cereal, or large amounts of butter and jelly on whole-grain bread *will* add empty calories and lead to weight gain.

SUGGESTED DIETARY GOALS

Americans seem to have a fairly clear idea of sound nutritional principles. What is lacking is an understanding of the consequences of nutrition-related diseases such as hypertension, diabetes, and arteriosclerosis and the "widespread and unfounded confidence in the ability of medical science to cure or mitigate the effects of such diseases once they occur" [7].

Once people begin to take more responsibility for what they eat, drink, and smoke, there may be less need for national dietary goals. In the meantime, the Senate Select Committee on Nutrition has adopted seven dietary goals with which everyone should be familiar [8].

Goal 1. To avoid overweight, consume only as much energy (calories) as expended. Decrease energy intake and increase exercise if overweight.

This goal is important because fifteen million Americans are overweight to the extent that it raises their risk of suffering from hypertension, diabetes mellitus, heart disease, and gallbladder disease. The best protection against heart disease may be weight reduction [9]. Overweight may be one of the most serious nutritional problems in America today.

Goal 2. Increase consumption of *fresh* fruits and vegetables and whole grains to 48 percent of food intake.

Fresh fruits and vegetables and whole grains furnish complex carbohydrates. Since 1910 there has been an *increase* in fat as an energy source in American diets, and a *decrease* in complex carbohydrates. Sugar—cane, beet, corn syrup, molasses, and honey—a simple carbohydrate, has replaced the more complex carbohydrates in fruits, vegetables, and whole grains. This change seems to be partly related to the relatively small amount of television advertising for complex carbohydrates as opposed to the intense promotion of sugar cereals, drinks, candy, ice creams, and so on. So, the food industry influences our choices, despite the fact that diets high in complex carbohydrates seem to reduce the risk of heart disease [10].

Goal 3. Reduce consumption of refined and processed sugars to 10 percent of daily intake.

The increase in the use of refined sugar is due in large part to the food industry's efforts to create foods that are competitive. For example, the addition of sugar to cereal was a direct result of a slump in cereal sales [11]. Some of the dangers inherent in high sugar intake are dental disease, increased requirement of certain vitamins such as thiamine, which are needed to metabolize carbohydrates, and increased burden on other parts of the diet to make up for the empty calories contained in sugar [12].

Goal 4. Reduce fat consumption to 30 percent of daily intake.

Since fat is the most concentrated form of food energy—9 calories per gram as opposed to 7 for alcohol and 4 for protein and carbohydrate—reduction in fat intake can influence weight control and obesity. Also, fat intake appears to be related to cancer of the breast and colon, and colon cancer correlates highly with meat consumption [13].

Goal 5. Reduce intake of saturated fat to 10 percent, and take in 10 percent of calories in polyunsaturated fats and another 10 percent in monounsaturated fats.

Goal 6. Reduce cholesterol consumption to 300 grams (g) a day.

Goals 5 and 6 are related because high levels of fat, saturated fat, and cholesterol occur most often in animal protein: meats, poultry, and fish. An increased use of vegetable protein will reduce the intake of saturated fat and cholesterol, as will eating lean meats, fish, whole-grain breads and cereals, sunflower, sesame, and pumpkin seeds, almonds, walnuts, peanuts, salad dressings made with polyunsaturated oils, skim milk, peas, beans, and lentils. On the other hand, it would be wise to try to *avoid*, or at least cut down, consumption of most cheeses and cheese spreads, except cottage cheese, tuna in oil, pork loin and butt, ground beef, whole milk, ice cream, ham, sockeye salmon (canned), dark turkey and chicken meat, and other foods that derive more than 30 percent of their calories from fat. What is most disturbing is that many of the following foods may contain a great deal of saturated fat: nondairy coffee creamers, convenience spreads, cookies, commercial snacks such as potato chips, baked goods, crackers, and mixes, and synthetic whipped creams or toppings. Until the government requires manufacturers to identify the type of oil used in these foods, it is recommended they not be consumed [14]. Since cholesterol is such a controversial subject, it will be discussed separately in a later section.

Goal 7. Limit intake of table salt (sodium chloride) to 5 g a day.

Salt consumption is estimated at about 6 to 18 grams a day per person, whereas the average requirement for sodium is about one-fourth a gram. Sodium occurs naturally in vegetables, and salt is added to most processed foods, so all requirements will be met without adding any salt in cooking or at the table. The desire for salt is not a physiological need but an acquired taste, and people should throw away their salt shakers if they want to move toward wellness.

Salt seems to be a factor in elevated blood pressure. There is some evidence that imbalance with potassium intake may be a factor. An alarming fact is that millions of children are moving toward hypertension (high blood pressure), and that taking too much table salt is a factor in some, if not most, of these cases. High salt intake also appears to be related to vascular disease, stomach cancer, cerebrovascular disease, and migraine headaches, and simply reducing the intake of salt can increase the length and quality of life for millions.

Some foods that should be avoided are olives, bacon, frankfurters, ham, salami, other salty meats, canned crabmeat, salmon, and tuna, chipped beef, all salted snack foods such as pretzels, nuts, crackers, and potato chips, seasonings that contain salt such as catsup, american cheese, monosodium glutamate [15], and any foods that taste salty or whose labels list salt as a chief ingredient.

VITAMINS

There is a growing concern that our diets may not supply all our nutritional needs, as a result of soil depletion, which produces crops that are nutritionally inferior, the increasing use of toxic insecticides, which leave harmful residues on food and kill important soil micro-organisms and earthworms, an increasing tendency to pick produce before it has ripened to its full nutritional state, an increasing use of chemicals and processing of food, an increasing intake of vitamin-free sugar as up to one quarter of daily intake, and the use of chemical additives that may be toxic and may be replacing other essential food elements. As early as 1943, the Federal Food and Drug Administration (FDA) realized that food processing was destroying important nutrients, and regulations were passed requiring commercial food companies to enrich their products. However, at that time, the FDA acknowledged that better nutrition could be ensured by natural foods, rather than by enrichment [16]. Because of this acknowledgement, we ought to be aware that "enriched" food, such as breads or cereals are *not* nutritionally equivalent to natural grains and cereals. All of these factors may be influencing our ability to obtain sufficient nutrients in our diet.

There may also be other conditions that lead to an increased need for vitamins. Some of these situations are: any difficulty with the digestive tract (for example, diarrhea, colitis, liver or gallbladder disorders); pregnancy; breastfeeding; increased physical activity; infections; the use of antibiotics, aspirin, estrogen, steroids, sulfa drugs, anticoagulants; inhaling polluted air, drinking polluted water;

and prolonged emotional stress [17]. In addition, heavy smokers, people with broken bones, those who are older and/or have poor eating habits or reduced gastric secretions, or those who drink have increased need for one or more of Vitamins A, B complex, and C [18]. Furthermore, all important nutritional elements have not yet been isolated and those that have been isolated have not been completely studied. For this reason, although food supplements may carry a statement such as: "need for in human nutrition is not established," this may be because the element has not been *studied* sufficiently, not that it may not be essential.

Signs of Vitamin Deficiency

Signs of vitamin deficiency vary individual by individual, and many of us walk around with subclinical deficiencies that have not reached the disease state but may be interfering with high-level wellness. One general clue to nutritional deficiency—that is, subclinical deficiency— is unhealthy skin or an unhealthy-looking mouth. There may also be some nonspecific complaints that could indicate nutritional or laboratory test signs, such as loss of appetite, anxiety, confusion, depression, fatigue, headache, insomnia, poor concentration, digestive upsets, palpitation, tingling or numbness in the fingers or toes, muscle pain or weakness, and irritability [19].

Since vitamin deficiencies manifest themselves in so many different ways and vary so person by person, each of whom is biochemically different from the other, many nutritional experts suggest that people experiment with vitamin usage—within recommended levels. Figure 2-1 gives a list of currently isolated vitamins, with their functions and sources, and with symptoms that may indicate deficiency in the particular vitamin. It would, of course, be foolhardy and possibly even dangerous to take vitamins impulsively and without adequate study and, if necessary, consultation with a nutritionally informed practitioner [20-33]. As a guide, Figure 2-2 shows the RDA or Recommended Daily Allowance [34-37].

MINERALS

Minerals play a vital role in body chemistry. Scientists continue to study the functions of minerals, but it is clear that a diet composed of large amounts of highly processed or refined foods and sugar cannot supply adequate minerals [38]. Including a wide variety of foods in the diet used to ensure an adequate intake. Today, "negative ecological trends, modern food processing, and changing food habits" [39] make it difficult to ensure an adequate mineral intake. Some minerals, such as calcium, magnesium, phosphorus, potassium, sodium, and sulfur, are required by the body in large amounts. Others, referred to as trace elements, are required in lesser amounts, but they are just as vital to wellness. Figure 2-3 gives information on minerals [40-50]; and Table 2-1 shows vitamin and mineral content for selected foods.

CHOLESTEROL

There is not a complete agreement on the subject of cholesterol. Since the original animal studies were completed, additional information has been learned. Even the early animal studies have been questioned by some experts who claim they were invalid because they were completed using rabbits who are natural vegetarians and who have no way of converting cholesterol to bile the way humans do. Secondly, the rabbits were fed purified cholesterol crystals, whereas cholesterol occurs in foods with its natural companion, lecithin [51].

A later finding was that cholesterol has two forms, a harmful one and a helpful one—LDL, or low-density lipoprotein, and HDL, or high-density lipoprotein. The level of LDL seems to be related to the consumption of cholesterol-rich foods, whereas HDL appears to be increased by exercising and by taking nicotinic acid (Vitamin B_3) [52]. LDL is harmful, but HDL appears to be protective of the heart. So, the higher the LDL cholesterol, the greater is the potential risk of heart disease, and the higher the HDL cholesterol, the more the heart is protected from disease.

This finding has not been as well publicized as the first, and consequently many people continue to reduce drastically their intake of food that contains cholesterol. This is unfortunate, since it is also a fact that the body produces *its own* cholesterol. Cholesterol is made into various body substances, including sex hormones and bile; bile itself is important in clearing the bloodstream of cholesterol. The body also has a feedback mechanism that adjusts total body cholesterol amount to the amount taken in through foods. When more cholesterol-rich food is eaten, the body manufactures less cholesterol. Also, blood cholesterol *can* increase due to other factors such as emotional stress [53].

Another important fact to remember is that lecithin can help dislodge cholesterol from blood vessels. Many cholesterol-rich foods *also* contain their own lecithin; for example, eggs contain *eight times* as much lecithin as cholesterol. Several experts say that eggs should not be avoided since they contribute so much to a healthy diet (see Figure 2-4). In the near-panic regarding cholesterol, people have deleted important nutrients from their diet, including lecithin, while trying to lower their cholesterol levels.

If you are concerned about your cholesterol levels, there are a number of things you can do. You can eat foods that contain lecithin, such as eggs or soybeans, and take lecithin granules (a supplement). Calcium seems to be effective in lowering cholesterol and strengthening heart muscle, so you can ensure adequate calcium intake. Vitamin C can help too; it seems to protect the walls of arteries so that cholesterol does not collect there. Vitamin E also protects the circulatory system, and improving circulation through active exercise is another way you can protect yourself. Magnesium seems to be helpful to the heart; calcium and magnesium intake can be increased by taking a dolomite supplement. Pectin is a food substance that limits the amount of cholesterol the body can absorb by lowering blood fats. Pectin is a natural carbohydrate found in fruits and vegetables and has none of the harmful side effects of cholesterol-lowering drugs; in addition, it does not interefere with the utilization of Vitamin A, as some drugs do. You can increase pectin in your diet by eating more oranges, bananas, cherries, grapes, pineapple, tomatoes, peaches, and raspberries. The best source is apples [54]—in the case of cholesterol, an apple a day (or better two) may keep the doctor away!

Other general wellness-enhancing measures will also keep cholesterol levels in balance. Diversifying meat intake, by eating more fish and poultry and less beef and pork, is a good idea. Cheese and eggs (especially eggs) should not be eliminated, since they are good sources of protein and other nutrients, and contain their own protection, lecithin. You should ensure an intake of one or two tablespoons of cold-pressed (not hydrogenated) vegetable oil daily and snack (lightly) on sunflower or sesame seeds. Refined sugar products— cakes, pies, ice cream, sweet rolls, and so on—ought to be eliminated, since they have few nutrients left in them after production and processing. Alcohol, too, should be eliminated since it increases triglycerides. Lastly, onions and garlic should be used liberally in cooking; they seem to affect cholesterol levels in a helpful way.

Table 2-1 Selected Foods and Their Vitamin and Mineral Content

	Minerals					Vitamins				
	Iron mg	Calcium mg	Phos- phorus mg	Potas- sium mg	Sodium mg	A mg	Thia- mine mg	Ribo- flavin mg	Nia- cin mg	C mg
1 glass milk or 1 container yogurt	.1	280	270	50	19	350	.08	.42	.1	2
1 cup green beans, cooked	.8	62	20	204	2	830	trace	.1	.6	16
1 cup broccoli spears, cooked	1.2	132	100	405	15	3,750	.14	.29	1.2	135
1 cup green peas, steamed	1.9	22	122	200	1	960	.3	.1	2.3	24
1 cup cooked spinach	4.0	167	33	470	74	14,580	.13	.25	1.0	50
½ medium cantaloupe	.8	25	64	910	40	6,540	.08	.06	1.2	63
1 cup cottage cheese	.9	207	360	170	625	430	.1	.6	.2	0
3½ ounces liver	9.0	8	476	380	184	53,400	.3	4.1	16.5	27

Food										
1 cup cabbage as cole slaw	.5	47	30	240	150	80	trace	trace	.3	50
1 cup grated carrot	.9	43	29	410	51	13,000	trace	trace	.7	7
1 cup steamed kale	1.3	130	57	260	29	8,000	trace	.2	.8	60
1 cup mustard greens, steamed	4.1	308	60	510	68	10,050	.1	.2	1.0	60
1 medium baked potato	.7	13	66	500	4	10	.1	trace	1.2	15
1 medium banana	.7	8	44	390	1	190	trace	trace	.7	10
½ grapefruit	.5	21	54	290	4	10	trace	trace	.3	72
1 cup brown rice	4.0	78	608	310	18	0	.6	.1	9.2	0
1 cup wheat germ	5.5	57	744	550	5	0	1.4	.5	3.1	0
½ cup sunflower seeds	3.5	60	418	460	15	0	1.8	.2	13.6	0
¼ cup (4 tablespoons) brewer's yeast	5.0	70	584	631	40	trace	5.2	1.0	12.9	0

Sources: *USDA Handbook*, 1975, p. 456.
USDA, *Nutritive Values of Food*, Home and Garden Bulletin No. 72, 1971.
Carolynn E. Townsend, *Nutrition and Diet Modifications*, Albany: Delmar, 1972, pp. 202–206.

FIBER

With the increasing processing and refinement of fruits, vegetables, and grains, the American diet is very low in fiber or roughage. It is thought that low-fiber diets may be related to the increase in lower bowel disease and cancer of the colon, because fiber seems to promote movement of food through the digestive system more quickly, decreasing constipation and the chance of absorbing toxic materials and cholesterol. Not all fibers are equally effective at all functions: apples, apple cider, and oatmeal are most useful for ridding the body of cholesterol, while wheat bran, whole grains, nuts, beans, fresh and dried fruits, and vegetables are more useful for maintaining bowel regularity.

Increasing fiber intake seems to be a good preventive measure, and it is even thought to be useful for those who already have bowel problems such as diverticulosis [55]. Increasing dietary fiber should be part of a lifelong pattern. One simple way is to scrub fruits and vegetables, rather than peeling them; another is to begin to take wheat bran daily. Plain, untreated bran can be purchased at health stores and in many supermarkets. Take one teaspoon of bran with each meal, working up to two teaspoons with each meal. Bran can cause some gas at first, but this will end shortly, and the substance causes no irritation to the bowel. One simple way of testing whether sufficient bran is being taken in is to increase bran very gradually until you can move your bowels without straining. Since bran is a natural food substance, there is no risk in taking it, whereas there can be risks in taking laxatives [56].

There are numerous bran cereals on the market, but many of these contain large amounts of sugar. It is easier—and cheaper—to buy plain bran and mix it with water, milk, or fruit juice, sprinkle it on oatmeal or other cereal, add it to soups, or bake it into bread or homemade dishes. Bran is too dry to eat plain, and in any case it should be taken with fluid since fiber holds water and additional fluids must be drunk when bran is taken. Bran also contains phytate—as do corn, rice, soybeans, and peanuts—and interferes with absorption of iron, calcium, zinc, and magnesium from the small intestine. Because of this factor, you may choose to consume bran between meals and/or make sure that you get additional amounts of the minerals mentioned [57]. As with any food substance, it is not wise to change the diet suddenly to include huge amounts of fiber. A gradual increase, while ensuring that several sources of fiber are taken in, is in line with a balanced approach to nutrition.

Another point to keep in mind is that plant fiber (cellulose) is not broken down in the digestive process. There is *no* enzyme that aids in the digestion of cellulose. Therefore, when you eat lettuce, celery, radishes, cucumbers, and so on, it is important that you break up the cellulose into very tiny pieces by chewing each bite extremely well. If this is not done, cellulose can lead to bloating and gas.

FOOD ALLERGIES

An allergy occurs when the body guards against the intrusion of a foreign substance; in this case, the foreign substance is a food. Just as vitamin and mineral deficiencies can trigger emotional reactions, so can foods, and people who suffer from unexplained mood swings or chronic depression may be allergic to one or more foods; when they have sought medical attention and are told, "All your tests are normal," they might begin to think they are neurotic. Although not all allergists acknowledge that allergies can cause depression, tension, and fatigue, many do. Sometimes individuals are mildly sensitive to a number of foods, and an allergy will only show up when they overeat the foods, eat several of the offending foods at once, or when their resistance is low because of colds or infections. Symptoms of food allergy vary; some to note appear in Figure 2-5. A problem-oriented approach is to become a detective, tracking down possible sources of food allergies. Figure 2-6 shows common sources of food allergy. Those who suspect an allergy can start by listing foods they hate or crave. Hating or craving foods often indicates an allergy or some type of food intolerance. If no foods can be eliminated this way, other steps can be taken [58]. Going to an allergist for skin patch tests is probably not the answer; many allergists consider these tests unreliable. A better strategy is to begin an elimination diet test. Eliminating milk, chocolate, and cola is a logical way to start this kind of test, but whatever the foods chosen it is crucial to understand that all products containing the foods must also be avoided during the test—and thereafter if the test proves conclusive—and that a constant lookout must be kept for hidden sources of the foods (see Figure 2-7). If individuals feel dramatically better after a week or two, it is pretty clear one (or all) of these foods caused the symptoms. To be certain, they can reintroduce the food(s) and see whether symptoms recur.

It may be helpful to keep a diary of symptoms for several days before beginning an elimination program. Some people may feel worse for several days when they begin an elimination test; this is due to "withdrawal" symptoms. Their bodies may miss the offending food. If the allergy is severe, it may take two or three weeks before relief occurs, but it is important to persevere.

If offending foods are carefully avoided for several months, it may be possible to eat that food again in small amounts without triggering a reaction. But people who have allergies should be aware that they can never again eat that food on a daily basis unless they are willing to endure allergic symptoms. They must restrict their intake of these foods to no more than once every four days. That way body tolerance levels will not be exceeded, and symptoms will probably not develop.

An additional way to test for food allergies is through the muscle strength test developed by Dr. John Diamond. He has developed a discipline called behavioral kinesiology. Body muscles are used as indicators of body energy. Dr. Diamond contends that the thymus gland (located in the middle of the chest where the second rib joins the breastbone) is the seat of Life Energy. The thymus produces cells that help resist infection and cancer and assists lymph to dispose of waste and toxic materials; it also seems to monitor and regulate energy flow, it can correct imbalance, and it is very sensitive to stress. Thus, one way of testing for food allergy—a stress or alarm reaction to foreign substances—is to use the muscle test. The deltoid muscle in the arm is used as an indicator of body energy and resistance to stress. If the deltoid should test weak (the person cannot hold his or her arm up while working against the push of another person's arm), the energy supply to the thymus is insufficient, or the gland is not active at that moment [59]. Some foods seem to drain energy from certain people. The following test can be used to test another person for the body's reaction to foods:

1. Have the person stand erect, right arm relaxed at the side, left arm held out parallel to the floor at shoulder height with elbow straight.
2. Face the other person and place your left hand on his or her right shoulder. Then place your right hand on the person's extended arm just above the wrist.
3. Tell the person you are going to try to push the extended arm down and ask him or her to resist with all possible strength.
4. Now push down on the extended arm firmly and quickly to test the spring and bounce.*

*© 1979 by John Diamond, M.D. *Behavioral Kinesiology*, Harper & Row.

Next, the test is performed again, this time with the other person placing a bit of a suspect food in his or her mouth and holding it there. If the muscle tests weak, ask the person to remove the food. If the muscle is strong, redo the test, asking him or her to touch the thymus with the right arm while holding the food in the mouth. (Foods that are extremely detrimental seem to lead to a weak muscle test, while those that are less detrimental may not lead to a weak muscle test until the thymus is touched.) Supplements and brands of foods can also be tested this way.

FOOD PRODUCTION, PURCHASE, AND PREPARATION

Many people refuse to accept the idea that soil quality affects food quality. Yet fertilizers do seem to influence the mineral composition of plants. For example, the iodine, zinc, cobalt, and selenium content of plants will vary, depending on the soil content of that mineral. In addition to loss of nutrients due to soil condition, some foods lose nutrients during storage and shipping, due to harvesting of unripe fruits and vegetables, soaking, pesticides, and chemicals and heat used in processing. Exposure to heat and light destroys some vitamins, and the freezing, canning, and refinement processes destroy more. Although refining processes replace *some* of the substances removed, they do not replace others, and there is bound to be an imbalance in the way they are presented to the body for use. Vitamins work in concert, and they have to be available in specific combinations and amounts in order to be used effectively by the body. Unfortunately, these combinations and amounts are not yet known about completely [60]. So, until more is known, it may be wisest to stick with the natural product and stay away from refined and processed foods and "ready-to-eat" products.

It is also wise to read labels carefully when buying processed foods. It is often safest to buy products that contain the fewest substances; labels that have a long list of additives, preservatives, fillers, mixes, stabilizers, and so on, are developed primarily with the producer in mind, not the consumer. In some states, and for some products, not all ingredients have to be listed on labels. For example, manufacturers use special codes that state how long processed foods remain fresh, but this information is not always available to consumers unless they know how to break the code. One source of information for consumers is available from the Consumer Protection Board (see Appendix, Wellness Resources). People should begin to question why they are willing to pay more for hamburger extenders than for hamburger, and why they buy artificial fruit flavors rather than real fruit. Supermarket shelves are filled with more and more formulated or engineered "foods." These "foods" have been developed to resemble real food, but often they consist mostly of chemical substitutes. Many of these foods have been developed strictly for "convenience or to develop a new taste in the consumer" [61]. It is useful to question the purchase and use of such nutritionally questionable items.

Besides steering clear of highly processed and refined foods, learn how to conserve nutrients that *are* available in the foods you purchase. Some principles to use are: refrigerate fresh foods immediately after purchase. Refrigerate oils so they do not become rancid. Check freezers to make sure they are at 0°F or lower. (Since most freezers do not reach this low temperature, storage times should be shortened.) Use very little water in cooking foods, and drink the reserve liquid, add it to the meal in some way, or use it in soup stock. Cook meats slowly at low temperatures (after destroying surface bacteria by cooking for 1 hour at 300°F). Eat raw foods as much as possible, cook potatoes in their skins, and leave beans and peas in their pods until cooking time. Buy small quantities of fresh foods to avoid storage losses. Cut produce into large pieces when cooking; the greater the exposed surface in cooking, the larger the loss of nutrients. Scrub produce rather than peeling, since the outer coat often contains nutrients and fiber.

INGESTION OF CHEMICALS

Protein is a nutrient all people need every day in order to be healthy. In the United States, people tend to eat too much protein, and much of it is excreted without being used. Unfortunately, much of the protein consumed is in the form of meat and of fish like trout, bass, perch, tuna, and swordfish. All of these are very high on the food chain. For example, cattle eat grain, and the fish mentioned are predators who eat other fish. Pesticides and toxic substances such as mercury are more heavily concentrated in the tissues of higher organisms. So, when people eat high on the food chain, they take in concentrated residues of pesticides and unsafe amounts of mercury. Since virtually all the pesticide residues accumulate in fat, the likelihood of taking in harmful chemicals can be reduced by choosing low-fat dairy products such as cottage cheese, low-fat milk, and yogurt, grains and cereals, potatoes, leafy and root vegetables, fruits, and legumes, by eating small nonpredatory fish, and by reducing the intake of beef. Since long-term studies of the effects of taking in these harmful chemicals have not been completed, it is difficult to know what effect they may have on our bodies [62]. It therefore seems sensible to avoid them as much as possible.

There are other chemicals individuals may be taking into their bodies without questioning their effect on wellness. Coffee, tea, cola drinks, cocoa, and other products that contain caffeine or theobromine or other stimulants rob the body of B vitamins and can lead to light-headedness, headache, irregular heartbeat, ringing in the ears, irritability, rapid breathing, nervousness, twitching, difficulty sleeping, and seeing light flashes. Both alcohol and stimulant drinks decrease wellness by placing the body in alternating highs and lows. Alcohol, too, is harmful to the body—damage to the liver and nervous system are just two problems it causes—and to infants born of mothers who drink. Also, people who take three or more alcoholic drinks daily have a higher rate of blood pressure [63]. Some suggestions for cutting down on alcohol consumption are given in Chapter 4; other sources of help are given in the Appendix. It may be easier to give up drinks that contain stimulants; some suggestions for this are given later in this chapter.

Still other sources of chemicals are food products that have chemicals added to enhance flavor or color when inexpensive food sources are used, to ensure consistency, or to control acidity or alkalinity. These chemicals are referred to as *additives*. Some of them are harmless (lecithin, ascorbic acid), while others may be risky to take in (nitrites, nitrates, monosodium glutamate or MSG, artificial colorings or flavorings, cellulose). In general, it is wise to keep informed about food additives, communicate your concerns about additives to government and industry, read package labels carefully, try to eat unprocessed and unrefined foods as much as possible, and take Vitamin C or drink orange juice prior to eating any food substance containing nitrites or nitrates. The one age group where more stringent measures may be needed are children. Dr. Ben Feingold has demonstrated that hyperactivity in children is frequently the result of artificial colors and flavors or other additives. He has developed a Kaiser-Permanente Diet that seems to reduce this problem. Since children are "notoriously unreliable" and may resort "to lying and stealing to fulfill their craving for forbidden foods" [64], parents who wish to use this diet may require additional counseling and assistance to overcome these problems.

People who smoke decrease their wellness by canceling out the helpful effects of vitamins and by increasing their risks of lung diseases. Although many people know these facts, they still find it difficult to stop smoking. Teenagers seem nonchalant about the harmful effects of smoking and use denial by saying, "It will never happen to me." Some adults also deny the reality of how harmful smoking is, or maintain that they choose not to live if they cannot obtain the pleasure they feel they get from smoking. One situation that often gives pause to smokers is the occurrence of pneumonia or lung cancer. Steps to take to end smoking appear in Chapter 7.

TIMES OF SPECIAL NUTRITIONAL NEED

It is important to be aware of stressful periods and the special nutritional demands of these times. Stresses in daily life, such as minor infections, trauma, pain, loss of sleep, anxiety, heat, heavy work, and inadequate carbohydrate intake require a 30 percent increase in protein consumption. There are individual differences, however, and these may increase this requirement. Probably the best way to judge whether adequate protein is being taken in and used by the body is the condition of nails, hair, and skin. Because they all require protein for growth, they are good indicators of adequate protein intake. You can also note whether burns, cuts, or scratches heal quickly; if they do not, additional protein may be needed.

Preschool children and pregnant and nursing women require added calories, protein, vitamins, and minerals. The elderly require diets where protein provides 12 percent of the total amount eaten. Older people may also require additional amounts of Vitamins A, D, B_{12}, and C, and thiamine, riboflavin, folic acid, calcium and iron [65].

Pregnant women need to be especially careful about drinking alcoholic beverages. There is an established link between birth abnormalities (growth deficiency, small head size, delayed mental growth, genital, heart, eye, and ear defects, disturbed sleep patterns, and extra fingers or toes) and drinking during pregnancy. Even one or two drinks could be dangerous. Pregnant women should be cautioned against drinking at all [66].

Pregnant women have increased needs for the following nutrients: Vitamin B_6 (to control swelling due to water retention), folic acid (to increase infant's resistance to illness and mental retardation, and to reduce toxemia, abruptio placenta, premature birth, afterbirth hemorrhaging), Vitamin C (to reduce leg cramps, to shorten labor, and to decrease pain, hemorrhage after delivery, and problems with urination), and Vitamin E (to protect the infant from hemolytic anemia) [67].

People who live in urban areas where there is a high ozone level may need to increase their intake of Vitamin D, since ozone absorbs the ultraviolet radiation from the sun which is needed to produce Vitamin D in the body. Other vitamins and minerals reported to reduce the toxic effects of particular pollutants are Vitamins A, B, C, E, calcium, iron, magnesium, manganese, phosphorus, selenium, and zinc; deficiencies of these substances have been found to add to the carcinogenicity of environmental pollutants [67].

Additional Vitamin A and protein seem to be needed when people are in contact with PCBs and some insecticides, such as dieldrin, Arochlor 1242, and DDT. Vitamin A also inhibits tumors in respiratory and reproductive systems, may protect against some of the dangers of cigarette smoke, and prevents precancerous tissues from turning cancerous. The diets of children, teenagers, pregnant women, and older people may not allow a proper margin of safety [68], and they certainly need Vitamin A supplementation to fight off the effects of exposure to toxic materials in the environment.

In addition to protecting people from some of the harmful effects of smoking, high doses of Vitamin C can prevent the toxic effects of arsenical compounds (used in the treatment of syphilis), cadmium, chromium, lead, mercury and mercurial diuretics, nitrates and nitrites, benzene, insecticides and insecticide residues, carbon monoxide, ozone, sulfates, x-rays, radioactivity, and radiation sickness.

People who must submit to x-rays can protect themselves somewhat by taking generous amounts of Vitamins C [69], P (bio-flavonoid), pantothenic acid (useful to reduce the effects of any stress), Vitamin B_6, and bee pollen [70]. The mechanism by which bee pollen reduces the effects of radiation is unknown, but one study reports both objective (increase in whole blood cells, serum protein, and gamma globulins) and subjective (less nausea, better appetite, better sleep patterns, less inflammation of treated areas) measures of wellness improved after bee pollen was administrated for the side effects of radium and cobalt 60 therapy for cancer of the neck of the uterus [71].

There are a number of dietary substances that offer protection against the effects of radioactive fallout of strontium 90 that is now found in leafy green vegetables, in milk, and in hard water. Each nuclear power plant and nuclear fuel processing plant releases radiation into the air. Even though regulatory agencies contend that these materials are of "negligible" amounts, radiation is cumulative, and damage from it is permanent [72]. It is its affinity for calcium (and bones) that makes strontium 90 so dangerous; it destroys the bone marrow. Kelp is a substance that binds most of the strontium within the intestine; then, together, they are both excreted. Kelp, or seaweed, comes from the sea and is at the bottom of the food chain, and thus it does not accumulate pollutants. It is a valuable food in other ways; it supplies carbohydrate (mannitol), fat, and protein, as well as some B vitamins, Vitamin C, and important minerals. Kelp is also a reliable source of iodine, which can protect from goiter and supplies rich amounts of potassium and magnesium; it also protects against synthetic female estrogens such as DES. In addition, iodine seems useful in improving precancerous breast conditions, such as dysplastic or abnormal changes in the tissue, nodules, benign tumors or cysts [73].

Kelp can be used as a salt substitute; it can be purchased dried (to use in cooking or salads) or in tablet or powder form. Treatment for radiation poisoning requires a large amount. According to the office of the Division of Biomedical and Environmental Research at The Atomic Energy Commission, a minimum intake of 10 g a day of alginate is needed; that is, one-third of an ounce, or several tablespoons [74]. To ensure that ample amounts of the substance reach all portions of the digestive tract, two generous tablespoons can be taken four times a day in some kind of thick soup, or six to eight tablets can be swallowed with milk four times a day.

Pectin, a substance found in apples, concord grapes, and in other fruits, provided they are unripe, also binds radioactive strontium and carries it out of the body. Two or three grated apples can be eaten three or four times a day, or one dozen pectin tablets can be chewed and swallowed three or four times daily. If neither algin nor pectin is available, three or four calcium or dolomite tablets can be taken four times a day.

Susceptibility to lead toxicity is decreased if children receive sufficient amounts of calcium, iron, phosphorus, protein, and Vitamins A, D, and C. Parents need to be appraised of this and take action to protect their children, especially those between 1 and 3 years of age, the peak years for lead toxicity [75].

Additional magnesium is needed to protect against the combined effects of the typical Western diet and fluoridated water. At least 6 mg of magnesium per kilogram of body weight is needed per day to maintain a healthy magnesium level in the body. However, people who ingest large amounts of protein, calcium, Vitamin D, and alcohol have an increased need for magnesium. If these individuals also drink fluoridated water, their need for magnesium increases further. So closely related are fluoride and magnesium, that the symptoms of magnesium deficiency are quite similar to those of fluoride toxicity: leg cramps, muscular twitching, convulsions, optical neuritis, and soft tissue calcification [76]. Magnesium also helps to prevent fat (lipid) deposits in the arteries and blood clot formation. Magnesium may have a protective effect against coronary heart disease. Women who take birth control pills have a lower serum magnesium level and faster clotting time; these women may be able to protect themselves somewhat from the harmful effects of "the pill" by taking additional magnesium.

Other trace minerals such as dietary chromium and manganese can protect against cardiovascular deaths. Chromium is difficult to find in foods, but one good source is dark brown or raw sugar; white sugar, in contrast, has had all the protective chromium removed during the refining process.

Miners who have been exposed to manganese dusts can develop toxic symptoms: a self-limiting psychiatric disorder and neurological changes. Miners with iron deficiencies are at high risk for manganese toxicity and need to take action to be protected [77].

People who are exposed to cadmium are at risk of developing damage to their reproductive processes and to unborn fetuses. Selenium has been demonstrated to protect against these effects as well as against toxic mercury levels. People who wish to eat tuna can protect themselves against the toxic mercury found in these fish by increasing their intake of selenium [78].

Zinc has been demonstrated to protect against cadmium toxicity. Higher levels of zinc can be taken to reduce the possibility of toxicity after exposure to cadmium.

Other situations that call for extra vitamins and minerals are listed in the sections on vitamins and minerals.

DIGESTING WELL

People who suffer from digestive problems after eating ought first to obtain a complete physical examination. Once serious problems have been ruled out, they can take action to deal with the situation themselves.

Overeating is perhaps the major cause of indigestion, bloating, and gas. Eating too much at one time overwhelms the digestive system and leads to food remaining overly long in the intestine because it cannot be digested properly. Changing food consumption patterns to six small meals a day will often eliminate gas problems and improve digestion, as will simplifying meals and combining fewer foods. Refined carbohydrates, especially white flour and sugar and foods made from them are often implicated in digestive disorders. Also, according to Devi [79], protein and carbohydrates should not be eaten at the same time since the latter start fermenting as the acid in the gastric juices affects the starch and creates gas and acidity. The same process can occur when starch—cereal, bread, rice, flour, corn, macaroni, and so forth—is eaten with foods that are acid—lemons, grapefruit, oranges, tomatoes, vinegar—or sulfurous—cabbage, peas, beans, cauliflower, brussel sprouts, or eggs. It is then preferable to eat foods in a sequence so that the citrus fruits and salads are eaten at the beginning of the meal, followed by neutral vegetables, such as beans, broccoli, celery, chard, eggplant, kale, peas, or peppers, followed by starch or protein.

Often, gas is due to a deficiency in hydrochloric acid or pancreatic enzymes. Restriction of protein intake to a six-hour period during the day might alone be sufficient to allow the pancreas to rebuild its supply of enzymes. Using cider vinegar (with oil for salad dressing), eating sauerkraut, buttermilk, and yogurt will often help the body rebuild important digestive secretions.

Eating overprocessed foods adds to the problem since they contribute to excess buildup of mucus in the small intestine, and nutrients are filtered out by the mucus. Pineapple or papaya may aid digestion, possibly by ridding the body of excess mucus.

Eating certain fruits together, for example, citrus fruits (lemons, oranges, grapefruit), melons (cantaloupe, watermelon), and bananas, is thought to lead to gas. To be on the safe side, people who have problems with gas should try eating these fruits separately, at different times of the day. For some individuals, nuts and seeds may be the only foods they can eat with fruits without starting a gas problem. Other causes of the problem can be eating cellulose—lettuce, celery, radishes, cucumbers, and so forth—without chewing each mouthful carefully and eating too quickly or in the midst of emotional turmoil.

There are a number of simple poses or exercises that can relieve gas pains. One is to lie flat on the abdomen, bending the legs at the knees in a relaxed way, and resting the upper body on the elbows. Mild, relaxed movement of the legs can further promote relief. Another pose to assume is the knee-chest position. In this pose, you kneel down, sitting on your heels. Then you lean forward, placing your elbows, lower arms, and hands on the floor in front of you (knees should be fairly close to chest). Headstands or a modified headstand are also useful. In the modified headstand, you bend "over the edge of a bed or padded table so the body forms a right angle, flexed at the hips, with the hands on the floor and the legs supported on the flat surface" [80].

LOSING WEIGHT THROUGH DIET

It is generally agreed that the healthiest way of losing weight is to change eating patterns by cutting down on or eliminating simple carbohydrates, such as cakes, cookies, sugar, or candy, reducing fat intake, and eating more complex carbohydrates such as fresh fruits, vegetables, and whole grains.

The first step, then, to reduce is to set up an intake record. Much overeating seems to be due to faulty feedback from hunger control mechanisms. Many overweight people seem unaware of how much they eat, and they may even claim that they never eat, yet they are surprised to see how much they are taking in when asked to keep a record of their food intake [81]. The following elements should be included in the intake record:

> the type and quantity of food eaten (calories *can* be included if you wish)
>
> the place where food is eaten
>
> the time food is eaten
>
> feelings right before eating
>
> the speed at which food is eaten
>
> social responses to eating

A notebook small enough to be carried at all times is useful for recording whatever is eaten. Figure 2-8 shows a way of recording this information.

You can keep a daily record for several weeks without trying to diet. Although no conscious effort is made to reduce at this time, weight may be lost as you begin to realize what you are eating and where and when, what feelings you may be covering up by eating, how quickly or unconsciously you may be eating, and how often social situations impinge on eating. It may also help if you visualize yourself as you want to be. You might say, "Close your eyes and picture yourself as a slim, confident person."

The next step is to set a realistic goal for weight loss, such as five to ten pounds. By setting realistic goals, you can learn to build success into your work. Once the initial goal is reached, a new one can be set. Goals that can be attained in a relatively short period of time provide motivation, whereas goals that require several months or a year to accomplish may result in frustration and failure. Weigh yourself regularly and chart your weight on graph paper to keep track of how you are progressing toward each goal. It is important that you weigh yourself at a set time on your weigh-in day, and in the same amount of clothes.

Once eating patterns are known and goals set, you can restructure your eating environment. There are specific instructions you can follow to make it more difficult to eat; reduce the number of times per day and the number of areas where eating occurs, make eating time only for eating, and increase energy output. Consider using the following suggestions:

1. Never go shopping when hungry.
2. Buy goods that require preparation before they can be eaten.
3. Prepare only enough food for one small portion.
4. Use small plates and shrimp forks.
5. Drink a glass of water before each meal.
6. Eat slowly, putting down the fork or spoon between each bite.
7. Use chopsticks if possible.
8. Chew each mouthful at least twenty times.
9. Place reminders to yourself in strategic places, such as pictures of your ideal self on the front door of the refrigerator.
10. Reward yourself with one of your favorite activities when you stick to your goal.
11. Stay out of eating areas (including the kitchen) except when eating or preparing food.
12. Eat only in one location each time you eat and only when sitting at the table; never eat standing up.
13. Turn off television, radio, and music when eating.
14. Concentrate only on chewing the food you are eating.
15. Leave the table as soon as you have finished your meal, and brush your teeth.
16. Park your car several blocks from where you work, and walk to your work or school area.

17. Get off the elevator one flight from where you are going, and walk the last flight.
18. Make a list of all the activities you enjoy (excluding eating); use one or more of these activities to reward yourself immediately when you have attained or shown improvement toward meeting your goal.
19. Every time you have an urge to eat, take a walk indoors or outdoors, or do a simple exercise.
20. Keep a jar full of cleaned, cut, uncooked vegetables; eat a handful of them if no other measure works to reduce your urge to eat. Some vegetables to use are: celery, carrots, green peppers, cauliflower, radishes, cucumbers, cabbage, mushrooms.
21. Stay away from refined, highly processed foods.
22. Tell family and friends, "I'm on a diet to lose weight, and I take responsibility for it, but please don't offer me food."
23. Every time you think of eating, block out the urge by thinking or saying the word, "stop."
24. Do not eat out at first; the food is too tempting.

ELIMINATING STIMULATING DRINKS

Use the suggestions below to eliminate your intake of stimulating drinks, such as coffee, tea, and colas.

1. Try drinking camomile tea or a hot carob drink.
2. Get sufficient sleep; the need for stimulating drinks may be due to body fatigue; pay attention to your body signals of fatigue.
3. Learn relaxing exercises, yoga, or meditation to reduce fatigue.
4. Increase intake of B vitamins to increase energy.
5. If possible, take a short midday nap, or at least sit or lie quietly for 5 to 10 minutes.
6. Observe daily fatigue patterns, and eat a high-protein meal before a sleepy period.
7. Try getting some fresh air and exercise at lunchtime.
8. Find a project that is meaningful; one that will enhance interest and alertness.
9. Be aware that there may be a withdrawal period, with increased fatigue, when you first stop drinking stimulants. A gradual cut-down may be best.

DEVELOPING A PERSONALIZED NUTRITION PROGRAM

Sensible eating patterns tend to be the exception. It is frequently difficult to eat properly while others around are eating potato chips and chocolate cake and guzzling scotch; they may also exert pressure to eat as they do, and consider a person who begins to avoid food additives, refined white sugar and flour, and other unhealthy foods as a "health nut." Besides, a correct diet almost always requires additional nutrition awareness, takes more time, and may be inconvenient.

Ease into eating that enhances wellness by moving slowly into a personalized nutrition program. For example, begin by adding two tablespoons of dry powdered milk to baked goods, creamed soups, pancakes, muffins, casseroles, cakes, and cookies. This one trick alone will provide additional protein, calcium, riboflavin, and several vitamins. Or start reducing your sugar intake by using part honey and part sweet fresh fruit; many fruits have a natural sweetness that makes sugar unnecessary. Buy or grow your own sprouts from soybeans, mung beans, alfalfa seed, or other beans. Sprouts are very low in calories and extremely high in Vitamins C, B_2, folic acid, B_3, pyrodixine, pantothenic acid, A, E, K, calcium, iron, phosphorus, and potassium. Seeds to sprout can be purchased in many supermarkets and health food stores; already sprouted seeds and beans can be found in produce departments of many supermarkets. Sprouts can be placed in salads, added to scrambled eggs and omelets (egg foo yung), used on top of soups, or added to rice.

Brewer's yeast or nutritional yeast can be purchased at health-food stores. Brewer's yeast is *not* baking yeast. Uncooked baker's yeast contains live yeast cells that are necessary for baked breads but threaten the body's use of B vitamins. When baker's yeast is cooked, it no longer interferes with B vitamins. Brewer's yeast is another kind of product, one that is low in fat and sugar and high in protein, vitamins, and minerals. There are now types available that are quite tasty. Since nutritional yeast *is* a unique taste, it can be introduced slowly by adding a tablespoon or two to soups, stews, breading for meats or vegetables, or hamburger mixtures. Wheat germ can be used to replace a half a cup (or more) of white flour in cooking, and it can be added to hot or cold cereals. Sunflower seeds can be eaten as a snack, or a handful or two can be added to meat loaf, bread, or salad. Since sunflower seeds are high in calories, a small amount should be used; even an ounce or two can provide important vitamins and minerals. Carob powder or chips can be substituted for chocolate in cakes, cookies, or hot drinks; carob is soothing and relaxing when placed in warm milk, and it is low in calories, naturally sweet, and high in protein [82].

An easy rule of thumb is that the potential for good nutrition increases the more you stay away from processed foods, sugar, fat, and salt, and the more you eat and drink fresh, uncooked fruits and vegetables and juices and eat whole grains and low-fat foods.

An important concept to remember is that the quality of food taken in determines the quality of life going on in each cell in the body. There is danger in becoming committed to a fad diet. It is more important to tune in to body messages that signal deficiencies or needs. On another level, it is important to become aware of how food is used as a substitute for comfort, love, relaxation, for release of tension or anger, for approval, or to deal with other uncomfortable feelings. Figure 2-9 provides an exercise that can facilitate this process.

Some suggestions that may be helpful to promote your health appear in Figures 2-10 and 2-11; Figure 2-12 can help you to assess your nutritional status.

You may think you have neither the time nor the energy to plan meals that meet all the requirements for normal and for stressful periods. In that case, you may wish to explore the use of supplements. There are hundreds of vitamin supplements available. Taking a few of the more popular vitamins may be unwise, since vitamins work together in concert. It is also unwise to assume that if a multivitamin is taken, all nutrients are provided in a scientifically balanced form. You can begin to examine labels critically to see that all vitamins and minerals are provided and that they are provided in correct potencies (refer to Figure 2-2). Read the labels of supplements carefully, note what is omitted and where "mcg" rather than "mg" are found, and compare prices. Often a supplement must be taken three times a day to supply the listed ingredients; 30 tablets of a good one-a-day supplement is about equivalent to 100 tablets of one that must be taken three times a day.

Be aware also that the way supplements are stored can affect their potency. Products are designed to keep their strength for six months to a year after opening. To ensure potency, vitamins should be refrigerated after being opened.

Although not all readers will be subjected to hospitalization, some will be. Those who are hospitalized should know the dangers of physician-induced (iatrogenic) malnutrition. Some of the practices that lead to malnutrition in hospitalized people have been summarized by Dr. Charles E. Butterworth, a physician [83].

1. failure to record the height and weight of those newly admitted to the hospital and to compare this with later weights—in one study reported by Dr. Butterworth, 61 percent of those studied lost an average of 6 kg (16 lbs) during hospitalization;
2. prolonged use of glucose and saline intravenous feedings with no food by mouth for a number of days;
3. withholding meals because of diagnostic tests;
4. diffusion of responsibility for care and rotation of staff at frequent intervals;
5. use of tube-feedings in inadequate amounts, of uncertain composition, and under unsanitary conditions;
6. ignorance of the composition of vitamin mixtures and other nutritional products;
7. failure to observe individual nutritional intake and to recognize increased nutritional needs due to injury, illness, and/or surgery;
8. performance of elective surgical procedures without first making sure that the patient is optimally nourished;
9. unwarranted use of antibiotics (and other medications that deplete nutritional reserves);
10. failure to appreciate the role of nutrition in prevention of and recovery from infection, trauma, illness, and surgery;
11. lack of communication between nutritionists, physicians (and nurses), and failure to take *each* patient's nutritional needs into account;
12. delay of nutritional support until patients are in advanced states of nutritional depletion, leading to irreversible conditions in some cases;
13. limited availability and use of laboratory tests to assess nutritional status.

Other factors that contribute to malnutrition in some hospital settings are: the increasing use of steam tables, and other food preparation procedures that deplete vitamins and minerals from food; the lack of fresh fruit and vegetables in hospital meals; the failure to personalize nutritional programs for those hospitalized *or* to assess their need for personalization; the failure to add nutritional coverage when patients are taking medications that deplete their protein, vitamin, or mineral status; the use of sugary desserts or snacks, fruit drinks, puddings, jello, cookies, and so on, which deplete vitamin and mineral reserves and add useless calories; the failure to add foods or supplements containing vitamins and minerals to promote wellness without the use of harmful or useless medications.

Patients should be aware of all these facts, and they can inquire regarding the nutritional program in their hospital, talk with their physician or nurse regarding their concerns, negotiate to bring their own food in, or plan some other action to ensure that their nutritional needs will be met.

Figure 2-1   Handy Reference to Vitamins: Functions, Deficiency Symptoms/Signs, Sources [20-33]

Vitamin	Functions	Deficiency symptoms or signs	Sources
A	helps fight infection, maintains cell wall strength, and prevents viruses from penetrating and reproducing; blocks production of cancerous tumors	night blindness, itching and burning of eyes, redness of eyelids, drying of mucous membranes, colds or respiratory troubles, dry rough skin, pimples or acne, susceptibility to eye infections, difficulty urinating or performing sexually	carrots, brocoli, kale, spinach, eggs, milk fat, fish liver oils, apricots, cantaloupes, organ meats*
B₁ (thiamine)	promotes appetite and good digestion, plays an important role in oxidation, blood and protein metabolism, and growth	tiredness with inability to sleep, swelling legs, loss of appetite, lack of enthusiasm, forgetting things regularly, aching or tender calf muscles, rapid heartbeat, overreacting to normal stress, constipation, feeling of going crazy	sunflower seeds, brewer's yeast, beef kidney,* whole-wheat flour, rolled oats, green peas, soybeans, beef heart, lima beans, crabmeat, brown rice, asparagus, raisins, desiccated liver, wheat germ
B₂ (riboflavin)	contributes to protein and carbohydrate metabolism, tissue repair and formation, growth in infants, proper nitrogen balance in adults, light adaption	feeling trembly, dizzy, or sluggish, burning feet, chapping lips, tiring easily, being overly nervous, having digestive disturbances, scaling of skin, having bloodshot eyes	beef, liver, kidney, or heart,* ham, chicken, hazelnuts, peanuts, hickory nuts, soybeans, soy flour, wheat germ and whole-wheat products, spinach, kale, peas, lima beans, brewer's yeast, sunflower seeds, eggs

	Function	Deficiency symptoms	Sources
B₃ (niacin)	dilates blood vessels, aids in carbohydrate metabolism and the use of Vitamins B₁ and B₂	having cold feet or body numbness, having a swollen bright red tongue or gums, feeling overly anxious, weak, or tired, having memory loss, developing prickly heat rash	wheat germ, wheat bran, brewer's yeast, salmon, prunes, lentils, chicken, peanuts, sunflower seeds, tuna, turkey, rabbit
B₆ (pyridoxine)	activates enzymes, aids in metabolism of fats, carbohydrates, potassium, iron, protein, and formation of hormones, nucleic acids, antibodies, hemoglobin, and lecithin, dissolves cholesterol and regulates water imbalance, may be useful in fighting off cancer, one form of anemia, and tooth decay	feeling tense, irritable or nervous, not being able to concentrate or sleep, having tics, tremors, twitches, bad breath, seborrheic dermatitis or eczema, bloating, puffiness, soreness, or cramping in menstruating or menopausal women	brewer's yeast, sunflower seeds, toasted wheat germ, brown rice, soybeans, white beans, liver, chicken, mackerel, salmon, tuna, bananas, walnuts, peanuts, sweet potatoes, cooked cabbage
B₁₂	maintains normal red blood cell formation and nervous system, aids in RNA and DNA manufacture, conversion of folic acid to folinic acid, carbohydrate, fat, and protein metabolism, fertility, and growth and resistance to germs	feeling apathetic, moody, forgetful, suspicious, soreness in arms or legs or having difficulty walking or talking, jerking of arms or legs	organ meats,* raw beef, clams, oysters, sardines, crab, crayfish, mackerel, trout, herring, eggs, some cheeses, nutritional yeast, sea vegetables (kombu, dulse, kelp, wakame), fermented soyfoods (tempeh, natto, and miso)

Figure 2-1 (continued)

Vitamin	Functions	Deficiency symptoms or signs	Sources
Folic acid	vital to blood formation, cell growth, synthesis of RNA and DNA, resistance to infections and to proper mental functioning	looking pale and wan, feeling "pooped," getting brownish spots on face and hands, panting with slight exertion	asparagus, desiccated or fresh liver,* fresh dark green uncooked vegetables, wheat bran, turnips, potatoes, orange juice, black-eyed peas, lima beans, watermelon, oysters, cantaloupe
Pantothenic acid	protects against environ-mental stress and infection, works with pyridoxine and folic acid to create anti-bodies, assists in production of body energy, protects against side effects of some antibiotics, aids in expelling trapped intestinal gas	having balky bowels, chronic gas or distention, feeling fatigued or not hungry, having constant respiratory in-fections, strange itching or burning sensations	soy flour, sunflower seeds, dark buckwheat, sesame seeds, brewer's yeast, peanuts, lobster, wheat bran, broccoli, mushrooms, eggs, oysters, sweet potatoes, cauliflower, organ meats*
Biotin	aids in metabolism of carbohydrates, proteins, and fats, assists in growth, maintenance of skin, hair, nerves, sebaceous glands, bone marrow, and sex glands	having poor appetite, sore mouth and lips, dermatitis, nausea and vomiting, de-pression, pallor, muscle pains, pains around the heart, tickling sensation in hands and feet	nutritional yeast, liver,* eggs, mushrooms, lima beans, yogurt, and a variety of nuts, fish, and grains

Inositol	not clear, but seems to be useful in controlling cholesterol level	not known	wheat germ, oranges, grapefruit, watermelon, peas, cantaloupes, whole-grain breads, and cereals, molasses, nuts, brewer's yeast, bulgar wheat, lima beans, oysters, peaches, lettuce, brown rice
Choline	essential to nerve fluid, liver functioning, keeping blood pressure down, increasing body resistance to infection	not known	egg yolks, soybeans, liver,* brewer's yeast, fish, peanuts, wheat germ, lecithin
C (ascorbic acid)	contributes to health of blood vessels, gums, teeth, and bones, essential to assimilation of iron, aids body in fighting off infection and cancer-producing substances and in normalizing blood cholesterol level, detoxifies some of the poisons due to smoking, aids in healing process, essential to collagen process, essential to collagen (body "glue"), slows down aging, and protects against stress	frequent bruises, poor healing, bleeding gums when toothbrushing, frequent infections, feeling run down, having an aching back due to disc lesions	green peppers, honeydew melon, cooked broccoli or brussel sprouts or kale, cantaloupes, strawberries, papaya, cooked cauliflower, oranges, watercress, raspberries, parsley, raw cabbage, grapefruit, blackberries, lemons, onions, sprouts, spinach, tomatoes, rose hip tea or powder

Figure 2-1 (continued)

Vitamin	Functions	Deficiency symptoms or signs	Sources
D	vital for maintaining health and growth of bones, for using calcium, and for metabolic functions affecting eyes, heart, and nervous system	weakness and generalized bone aches, localized back pain on arising or bending over, pain in areas where spinal vertebrae may have collapsed, brittle bones that break easily, pain in mid- to lower back	fish liver oil, Vitamin-D-enriched milk, eggs, salmon, tuna
E	seems to be useful in any condition where there is actual or threatened clotting, decrease in blood supply, increased oxygen need, externally when there are burns, or sores to heal, or to protect against exposure to radiation	not known	nutritional yeast, wheat germ, peanuts, outer leaf of cabbage, leafy portions of broccoli and cauliflower, raw spinach, asparagus, whole-grain rice or wheat or oats, cold pressed wheat germ, cottonseed, or safflower oil
K	essential to blood clotting	some types of bleeding without clotting	spinach, cabbage, cauliflower, tomatoes, pork liver,* lean meat, peas, carrots, soybeans, potatoes, wheat germ, egg yolks

*Remember: Any chemicals ingested by animals concentrate in their organs and especially their livers; if you decide to eat organ meats to ensure adequate intake of vitamins, you might consider taking extra amounts of the vitamins that detoxify your body, such as Vitamin C and pantothenic acid.

Figure 2-2 RDAs of Vitamins; Reasons Supplementation May Be Needed [34-37]

Vitamin	RDA	Reasons supplementation may be needed
A*	Adults: 5,000 I.U. daily Nursing mothers: 4,000 I.U. daily Pregnant women: 6,000 I.U. daily Children over 12: 4,500–6,000 I.U. daily Children under 12: 1,500–3,500 I.U. daily	Americans are eating 30 pounds less fresh fruit and 20 pounds less vegetables per capita per year than in 1950; cooking dramatically decreases the value of the vitamin; widespread use of fertilizers and pesticides interferes with body's ability to convert carotene into Vitamin A; high-protein diets require more Vitamin A to process; cold temperatures, air pollution require additional amounts of the vitamin.
B₁	1.2–1.5 mg daily	Cereal and rice producers remove thiamine when germ and outer coating is removed; large quantities are lost in cooking water; people who eat little or no organ meats, fresh vegetables, oatmeal, potatoes, and beans may receive little thiamine, as do people who have diarrhea, who eat excess sugars or carbohydrates, drink coffee or alcohol, take antibiotics, or smoke, and those exposed to stress or aging processes.
B₂	1.6–1.8 mg daily	Supplements are needed by people who eat snack foods, processed desserts, or commercial baked goods; the vitamin is destroyed by cooking or when antibiotics or oral contraceptives are taken; it is destroyed when milk bottles or meat containers are left exposed to light.

Figure 2-2 (continued)

Vitamin	RDA	Reasons supplementation may be needed
B_3	18–20 mg daily	Heavy intake of highly refined and/or carbohydrate foods requires more B_3 to metabolize; it is lost during cooking; its metabolism is interfered with when taking oral antibiotics; illness and taking alcoholic beverages decreases its absorption.
B_6	Adults: 2 mg daily Nursing and pregnant women: 2.5 mg daily	Losses of B_6 are due to refining, cooking, processing, storing, and to eating a high-protein diet; there is an increased need when taking steroids (such as cortisone and estrogen), oral contraceptives, or when pregnant or menstruating.
B_{12}	2 micrograms (mcg) daily	When eating only vegetarian meals.
Folic acid	400 mcg daily	Needed during pregnancy, when taking oral contraceptives, when growing or aging, when faced with trauma, infection, or chronic daily stress, or when drinking alcoholic beverages.
Pantothenic acid	10 mg daily	Needed to supplement processed food; greater need when subjected to infection, environmental stress, x-rays, surgery, or antibiotics.
Biotin	300 mcg daily	Needed when eating raw eggs or taking antibiotics or sulfa drugs or when eating beef (cattle are routinely given antibiotics and hormones).
Choline	non established yet	Infants need it if not breastfed (cow's milk does not contain this vitamin, but breast milk does).

C	30–45 mg daily	Needed to slow down aging processes, increase healing of infection, disease, or injury; decreases effects of toxic chemicals in the environment; if taking aspirin, more of this vitamin is needed; when smoking or drinking, more is required; soaking vegetables and fresh fruits in water or exposing fruit or juices to air destroys this vitamin.
D*	400 I.U. daily	Calcium is not absorbed without sufficient Vitamin D; needed at times of insufficient sun exposure in winter, when soot and air pollution filter out sun rays, when spending long hours in offices or indoors; when taking steroids, or when smoking.
E	30 I.U. daily	When outer leaves of vegetables are not eaten; when vegetables are placed in vigorously boiling water to cook (rather than bringing the water to a boil); when eating processed foods, exposed to smog, drinking chlorinated water, undertaking strenuous exercise, when exposed to air purifiers, static electricity, sun, x-rays; by those who take oxygen as a therapeutic measure, have had a heart attack or burn.
K	no requirement	People who are elderly, women with prolonged menstruation, people with liver disease, diarrhea, colitis, or who take antibiotics or anti-coagulants (blood-thinners).

*Note: Vitamins A and D are the only two vitamins that can be toxic if taken in excess; extra amounts of other vitamins are excreted by the body. If you note symptoms of overdosage in Vitamins A or D, discontinue taking it until symptoms disappear, then take a smaller dose.

Symptoms of Vitamin A overdosage: bone or joint pain that comes and goes, fatigue, insomnia, loss of hair, dryness and fissuring of lips, loss of appetite, peeling and flaking of skin, dizziness.

Symptoms of Vitamin D overdosage: nausea, weight loss, loss of appetite, head pain, calcification of bones, and in children a reduction in growth rate [35].

Figure 2-3   Handy Reference to Minerals, RDAs, Functions, Sources, Factors Leading to Insufficient Intake [40]

Mineral	Functions	Sources	Factors leading to insufficient intake
Calcium RDA: 1000 mg/day; 1.4 g for menopausal women	Keeps body framework rigid and teeth strong; creates tranquility in nervous system and calms nervousness; necessary for transmission of nerve impulses and for muscle contraction, clotting, some enzymes, "glue" (collagen) that holds body together and cells in place, and to regulate transport of substances in and out of cells	milk, cheese, eggs, green leafy vegetables, fish, butter, tomatoes, lean beef, whole wheat bread, yogurt, canned sardines, molasses, dolomite, soy milk, buttermilk	dieting to restrict calories or cholesterol; eating snack foods; drinking soft drinks; having a high protein intake
Magnesium RDA: 350 mg/day	Works with calcium to ensure good muscle movement and a strong heart beat; seems to prevent blood vessel and heart disease	whole-grain bread and cereals, fresh peas, brown rice, soy flour, wheat germ, nuts, swiss chard, figs, green leafy vegetables, citrus fruits, dolomite	having diarrhea, vomiting, taking diuretics, drinking soft water, eating processed foods

	Works/Function	Sources	Risk factors / Depletion
Potassium RDA: none, estimated need: 2.5 g/day for adults; .98 to 3.9 g/day for children	Works in concert with sodium to move materials through cells walls (osmosis) and maintains acid-base balance; helps muscles contract, heart to beat regularly, nerves to carry impulses properly, and food to be turned into energy	shredded raw cabbage, bananas, turkey, apples, fresh apricots, cooked broccoli, baked potato, wheat germ, molasses, spinach, dried fruit, fresh fruits and vegetables of all kinds	using convenience foods and highly processed foods; profuse sweating; taking certain diuretics (water pills) to lose fluid; taking cardiovascular drugs, steroids, laxatives, enemas; eating licorice candy; breastfeeding, having depression or ulcerative colitis
Selenium RDA: 50–200 mcg/day	Protects against heart disease and cancer; detoxifies the body from effects of pollutants and radiation; important for healthy skin and hair and for production of sperm cells	high protein foods such as meats, seafoods; whole-grain breads and cereals; brewer's yeast; asparagus, garlic, mushrooms	eating beef fed on corn or eating grains grown in selenium-poor soil (northeast, Florida, parts of Washington and Oregon, parts of the midwest); exposure to industrial pollutants
Manganese RDA: none established; estimate 2.5–7 mg/ day needed	Important to fat metabolism, bone formation, brain function, reproduction, and may protect against cancer of the pancreas	nuts, seeds, whole grains, fruits and vegetables, dry beans and peas, oatmeal	high levels of calcium and phosphorus diminish absorption of manganese

Figure 2-3 (continued)

Mineral	Functions	Sources	Factors leading to insufficient intake
Chromium RDA: none established; no estimate available	Helps to keep blood sugar levels in check	brewer's yeast, wheat germ, calf's liver, black pepper, and animal proteins except fish	refinement of cereal and grain products remove chromium; the elderly and those who are pregnant or protein-calorie malnourished are at risk for deficiency
Zinc RDA: 10–15 mg/day	Necessary for adequate breathing and digestion; important to taste, hearing, smell, appetite, normal growth and sexual functioning and reproduction, wound healing, healthy hair, good complexion; decreases lead toxicity	oysters, herring, liver, eggs, nuts, wheat germ and red meats	exposure to lead in gasoline, paints, joints in food cans, lead dust, drinking water that comes through lead pipes; eating canned tomatoes in quantity; foods containing phytate (beans, whole grains, and peanut butter) or calcium interfere with zinc absorption; being a vegetarian; regularly eating imitation meats, fast foods, white bread, fried potatoes, and rich desserts; drinking alcohol; being pregnant; having a cold or chest infection, kidney disease, heart problems, cancer, or taking birth control pills

Mineral	Function	Sources	At risk
Iron RDA: 10 mg/day	Works with copper to produce hemoglobin, an essential substance that carries oxygen to and from the body	organ meats, red meats, kidney beans, molasses, egg yolk, whole-grain breads and cereals	infants remaining on milk for long periods of time or those who are born of women who have low stores of iron; women who are menstruating, pregnant, breastfeeding or postmenopausal
Iodine RDA: 130–150 mcg/day	Necessary for normal functioning of thyroid gland; may protect against breast cancer	seafood, brown rice, beans, bananas, green leafy vegetables, kelp	living in areas where soil is low in this mineral (Great Lakes and Rocky Mountain regions)
Phosphorus RDA: 800 mg/day	Helps form nucleic acids; a component of cell membranes; aids in metabolism and storage and release of energy; a component of B vitamin coenzymes	liver, yogurt, milk, brown rice, wheat germ, sunflower seeds, brewer's yeast, meat, seafood, nuts, eggs, peas, beans, lentils	people with kidney disease; taking high doses of antacids
Sodium RDA: not established	Maintains osmotic pressure in the fluid outside the cells	celery, carrots, beets, cucumbers, string beans, asparagus, turnips, strawberries, oatmeal, cheese, eggs, coconut, black figs	some kidney and adrenal diseases; diarrhea; vomiting

Figure 2-3 (continued)

Mineral	Functions	Sources	*Factors leading to insufficient intake*
Sulfur RDA: not established	Part of the structure of amino acids, such as keratin, the protein of the hair; component of thiamine and biotin (vitamins); required for many oxidation-reduction reactions and coenzymes; contained in blood and other tissues; detoxifying agent; part of material found in skin, bones, tendons, and cartilage	cabbage, peas, beans, cauliflower, brussel sprouts, eggs, horse-radish, shrimp, chestnuts, mustard greens, onions, asparagus	no information available

Figure 2-4 Foods to Eat to Enhance Wellness

Eat these often	Vitamins provided	Minerals provided	Other advantages
Raw spinach*	A$_1$, B$_2$, C, folic acid, E, K	calcium, magnesium, potassium, copper, iodine, manganese	provides fiber and complex carbohydrate
Wheat germ (toasted)	B$_1$, B$_2$, B$_3$, B$_6$, inositol, choline, E	magnesium, potassium, chromium	high protein
Brewer's yeast	B$_1$, B$_2$, B$_3$, B$_6$, B$_{12}$, pantothenic acid, biotin, inositol, choline, E	selenium, chromium copper, zinc, magnesium, calcium, potassium	can be sprinkled on foods or in drinks
Kale	A, B$_2$, C	calcium, magnesium, copper, iodine, manganese	provides fiber and complex carbohydrate
Cantaloupe	A, folic acid, inositol, C	manganese	provides fiber and is a good dessert substitute for "sweets"
Sunflower seeds	B$_1$, B$_2$, B$_3$, B$_6$, pantothenic acid	manganese	easy to carry for a quick snack

*Spinach contains oxalic acid that can decrease the amount of available calcium, so be sure to eat enough calcium from other sources to make up for this.

Figure 2-4 (continued)

Eat these often	Vitamins provided	Minerals provided	Other advantages
Brown rice	B_1, B_6, inositol	magnesium, iodine	inexpensive, good source of protein when combined with beans, eggs, or milk products
Broccoli	A, folic acid, pantothenic acid, C, E	calcium, magnesium, potassium, copper, iodine, manganese	provides fiber and complex carbohydrate
Eggs	A, B_2, B_{12}, biotin, choline, D, K	calcium, iron, potassium	best source of all essential amino acids; low fat
Chicken (no skin)	B_2, B_3, B_6	copper, chromium	low fat; very usable protein
Whole grains	B_1, B_2, B_{12}, biotin, inositol, E	calcium, magnesium, iron, selenium, manganese, chromium	provides fiber
Wheat bran	B_3, folic acid, pantothenic acid		excellent laxative

Food	Vitamins	Minerals	Benefits
Peanuts (un-salted, no oil)	B_2, B_3, B_6, pantothenic acid, choline, E	copper, manganese, magnesium	complete protein when combined with a milk product
Cauliflower	pantothenic acid, C, E, K	manganese	provides fiber and complex carbohydrate
Peas	B_2, inositol, K	magnesium, manganese	low calorie, complex carbohydrate
Lima beans	folic acid, biotin, inositol, B_2	manganese	complex carbohydrate
Grapefruit	inositol, C	magnesium, manganese	low calorie, complex carbohydrate, corrects acid imbalance
Soybeans	B_1, B_2, B_3, choline, K	manganese	inexpensive source of protein
Asparagus	B_1, folic acid, E	manganese	low calorie, complex carbohydrate
Cabbage	B_6, C, E, K	potassium	low calorie, complex carbohydrate
Carrots	A, K	potassium, manganese	low calorie, complex carbohydrate
Fish	B_3, B_6, B_{12}, biotin, choline	calcium, zinc, copper, selenium	low fat, highly usable protein
Yogurt (plain)	D	calcium	high protein, low fat, provides helpful bacteria
Sprouts	A, B_2, B_3, folic acid, pyridoxine, pantothenic acid, E, K	calcium, iron, phosphorus, potassium	low calorie, inexpensive, high protein

Figure 2–5   Symptoms of Food Allergy

---

dark circles or puffiness under eyes

headache, some migraine

dizziness

bouts of sneezing

coughing when laughing or exercising

canker sores

diarrhea

rubbing the nose upwards

itching skin

irregular menstruation

sensitivity to light, sound, or cold

poor appetite

excessive perspiration

pale, sallow look

frequent or persistent colds

stomachache

low-grade fever

numbness or tingling

violent outbreaks

restlessness, insomnia

excessive throat mucus

excessive bowel mucus

excessive drooling

muscle aches

joint aches or swelling

bed-wetting

frequent urination

inability to concentrate

swollen hands, feet, face

tender, sore skin

tiredness after naps or eating

irritability

depression

behavior problems

clucking throat sounds

mottled tongue

sudden weight gain (5 pounds or more in one or two days)

Figure 2–6 /// 65

Figure 2–6 Common Sources of Food Allergy

milk	black pepper
chocolate	cloves
cola	onion
peanuts and other legumes	garlic
citrus fruits	coffee
corn	chicken livers
wheat	pickled herring
eggs	alcohol, especially red wines and champagne
pork	
beef	aged or strong cheese, especially cheddar
sugar	
fish and shellfish	cured meats such as hot dogs, bacon, and ham
tomatoes	food additives (BHA, BHT, sodium nitrate, salicylates, bleaching chemicals, chlorine)
mustard	

Figure 2-7   Foods To Avoid in Cases of Allergy to Milk, Wheat, Eggs, or Corn

Sources of milk	Sources of wheat	Sources of eggs	Sources of corn
cheeses	wheat breads	bread	corn-on-the-cob
ice cream	rolls	cakes	canned or frozen corn
sherbet	crackers	creamed pies	cornstarch
creamed soups	wheat cereals	custards	cornmeal
milk puddings	luncheon meats containing	french toast	popcorn
gravies	cereal fillers	ice cream	dextrose
sauces	breaded meats	icings	cough syrup
breads	cakes	meringue	creamed pies and cakes
cakes	pies	macaroons	corn oil
cookies	cookies	noodles	cornbread
medications using	doughnuts	pancakes	ice cream
lactose as a filler	gravies	mayonnaise	paper plates and cups
any products whose	macaroni	eggnog	corn syrup
labels contain the words:	dumplings	egg noodles	catsup
lactose, caseinate,	beer	hollandaise sauce	pasta
casein, lactalbumin,	gin	candies made with eggs	glue on stamps and
curds, and whey	whiskey	soups with egg or egg noodles	envelopes
	pretzels	puddings	
	hamburger mixes	souffles	
		products whose labels read:	
		albumin, vitellin, livetin, yolk,	
		powdered or dried egg globulin,	
		ovomucoid, or ovomucin	

Figure 2-8 My Eating Patterns for One Day

What I ate and drank	Place I ate it	Time eaten	What I was feeling at the time	How fast I ate and drank it	What else was happening at the time
coffee with cream and sugar	standing up in kitchen	7:00 a.m.	rushed	quickly	kids screaming in hallway
coffee with cream and sugar	at work	8:30 a.m.	worried about report I had not completed	can't remember	I was nibbling on a danish
coffee with cream and sugar	during break at work	10:00 a.m.	that I needed a pick-me-up	in a hurry	talking with friend, Irma
tuna fish salad on toast, coke, french fries	in cafeteria	noon	famished	can't remember	lots of noise and smells of food
candy bar	in hallway	2:00 p.m.	that I needed a pick-me-up—guilty	greedily	boss came in right before to ask for the report
coffee with cream and sugar	at desk	3:30 p.m.	tired	can't remember	talking on the phone, trying to get authorization for expense account

Figure 2-8 (continued)

What I ate and drank	Place I ate it	Time eaten	What I was feeling at the time	How fast I ate and drank it	What else was happening at the time
couple slices of salami	while cooking	6:00 p.m.	preoccupied with bad day at work	can't remember	kids fighting
macaroni and cheese casserole, frozen broccoli with breadcrumbs, apple pie à la mode	at dining room table	6:15 p.m.			
buttered popcorn, and coke	while watching television	8:30 p.m.	empty	can't remember	kids changing television channels

Figure 2-9 /// 69

Figure 2-9   I and Food

Directions:

Check "yes," "no," or "sometimes" for each of the sentences below. Go back when you have finished the exercise and think about whether you might wish to change your behavior or thinking related to each statement, and how you might go about doing so.

		Yes	No	Some-times
1.	I only use food to nourish my body	......	......	....
2.	Food is the only thing that can calm me down when I've had a rough day	......	......	....
3.	I use food when other people don't give me approval	......	......	....
4.	When I am at work or school, I get the urge to eat when things get tense	......	......	....
5.	I find myself eating greedily when I'm not even hungry	......	......	....
6.	I find myself eating and my mind is a million miles away	....	......	....
7.	I eat the way I do because that's the way my parents ate	......	......	....
8.	I eat even when I'm not hungry, just to be social	......	......	....
9.	I eat when I am bored and can think of nothing else to do	......	......	....
10.	I eat when commercials on radio, television, or the movies tell me I'm hungry	......	......	....
11.	I eat when the clock says I should eat	......	......	....
12.	I eat very quickly	......	......	....
13.	I eat "on the run"	......	......	....

Figure 2-10   Eating to Promote Health

Directions:

Sit down in a quiet place and plan a day's menu by asking yourself, What does my body need to enhance wellness? (Figure 2-9 may be useful in this process.) Think about what you have a "taste" for and how you might eat these foods or substitute healthier foods to assuage your hunger. When shopping, go to a store where you feel comfortable and relaxed. Take time to choose food; smell it, feel it, read the contents of cans and boxes carefully. Prepare the food in a relaxed manner. Smell the food, feel it, taste a very small bite of it, and observe what happens to a fruit or vegetable when you cut it. Notice how fresh and alive uncooked fruits and vegetables look. Pause before sitting down to eat, making sure you are relaxed. Clear your mind of tension and thought. Concentrate on what you are about to eat. Ask yourself, "Am I hungry?" If you find you are not, ask yourself, "Why am I eating now?" If you decide to go on eating, ask yourself how you are reacting to the food as you eat it—do you feel sad, contented, invigorated, harried, anxious, disappointed, indifferent? Notice the texture, temperature, taste, and smell of the food. Tell yourself, "This food is going to each cell in my body." Ask yourself, "Do my body cells need any more of this particular food?" Chew the food well, and notice the sensation of the food against your teeth and gums. Notice how fast or slowly you are eating. Adjust your rate so you feel comfortable and relaxed. Keep your mind focused on what you are eating.

Figure 2-11 /// 71

Figure 2-11   Designing My Diet Plan

Directions:

Ask yourself the following questions. Then use the information to design a customized diet for yourself, one that is not focused on temporary restrictions but on long-term enhancement of wellness.

1. What are my activity levels and how should I plan to include foods that meet my needs?

2. What are my past eating patterns?

3. Which of my past eating patterns do I wish to keep, and which do I want to change?

4. How do psychological factors (such as my feelings, tastes, preferences, need for variety) need to be planned for?

5. How does the amount of money I have for food fit into my diet to enhance wellness?

6. What barriers inside or outside me interfere with my designing a wellness-enhancing diet?

7. How can I overcome these barriers?

8. What other factors, unique to me, influence my diet planning?

Figure 2-12   Some Signs of Good Nutrition

---

alertness and responsiveness

shiny, lustrous hair

healthy scalp

thyroid gland of normal size

eyes that are clear and bright

lack of circles or puffiness around eyes

moist lips of good color

pink tongue with papillae present

pink, firm gums

clean, straight teeth with sufficient space between them

smooth, slightly moist skin

flat abdomen

well-developed legs and feet

lack of tenderness, weakness, or swelling in legs or feet

normal weight for height, age, and body build

erect posture, with straight back, arms, and legs, abdomen in, and chest out

well-developed, firm muscles

good attention span

lack of crying with ease, irritability, or restlessness

good appetite and digestion

elimination that is easy and regular

good endurance

high level of energy

good sleep pattern

NOTES

1. Roger J. Williams. *Nutrition Against Disease: Environmental Prevention.* New York: Bantam, 1973, pp. 3-4.
2. Select Committee on Nutrition and Human Needs. United States Senate. *Dietary Goals for the United States,* 2nd edition. Washington, D.C.: U.S. Government Printing Office, 1977, p. xxviii.
3. Frances Moore Lappe. *Diet for a Small Planet,* revised edition. New York: Ballantine, 1975, pp. 62, 78.
4. Ibid., p. 62.
5. Ibid., p. 81, 95-117.
6. Ibid., p. 62, 83.
7. Select Committee, *Dietary Goals,* p. xviii.
8. Select Committee, *Dietary Goals.*
9. Ibid., p. 7.
10. Ibid., p. 14.
11. Ibid., p. 31.
12. Ibid., p. 31-32.
13. Ibid., p. 38.
14. Ibid., p. 48.
15. Ibid., pp. 49-51.
16. Federal Food and Drug Administration. *Federal Register.* July 1, 1943a.
17. Charles Gerras, ed. *The Complete Book of Vitamins.* Emmaus, Pa.: Rodale, 1977, p. 9.
18. "Vitamin underachievers," *American Journal of Nursing* 78, no. 6, pp. 954-955.
19. Gerras, *Complete Book of Vitamins,* p. 20.
20. Ibid.
21. "Retinoids block phenotypic cell transformation produced by sarcoma growth factors," *Nature* 276: no. 16 (1978), pp. 272, 274.
22. Gerras, *Complete Book of Vitamins,* pp. 193-199, 213.
23. Rudolf Ballentine, *Diet and Nutrition, A Holistic Approach.* Honesdale, Pa.: 1978, pp. 157-222.
24. J. DeCosse et al. "Effect of ascorbic acid on rectal polyps of patients with familial polyposis," *Surgery* 78 (1975), pp. 608-612.
25. J. DeCosse, R. Condon, and M. Adams. "Surgical and medical measures in prevention of large bowel cancer," *Cancer* 40 (1977), pp. 2549-2552.
26. J. U. Schlegel et al. "The role of ascorbic acid in the prevention of bladder tumor formation," *Journal of Urology* 103 (1970), p. 155.
27. E. Cameron and L. Pauling. "Supplemental ascorbate in the supportive treatment of cancer: prolongation of survival times in terminal human cancer," *Proceedings of the National Academy of Sciences USA* 73 (1975), pp. 3685-3689.
28. S. Turley, C. West, and B. Horton. "The role of ascorbic acid in the

regulation of cholesterol metabolism and in the pathogenesis of atherosclerosis," *Atherosclerosis* 24 (1976), pp. 1-18.

29. E. Ginter. "Cholesterol: vitamin C controls its transformation to bile acids," *Science* 179 (1973), pp. 702-704.

30. J. Davies, P. Ellery, and R. Hughes. "Dietary ascorbic acid and lifespan of guinea pigs," *Experimental Gerontology* 12 (1977), pp. 215-216.

31. H. N. Londer and C. E. Myers. "Protective effect of vitamin E," *American Journal of Clinical Nutrition* 31, no. 4 (1978), p. 705.

32. Gerras, *Complete Book of Vitamins.*

33. "Are your deficiencies showing?" *Prevention* (March 1971), pp. 105-106.

34. Thomas Moore, "Pharmacology and toxicology of vitamin A," *The Vitamins*, Vol. 1. New York: Academic Press, 1967, p. 102.

35. Roseanne Howard and Nancie Herbold. *Nutrition in Clinical Care.* New York: McGraw-Hill, 1978, p. 87.

36. Leonard Newman et al. "Riboflavin deficiency in women taking oral contraceptive agents," *The American Journal of Clinical Nutrition* 31, no. 2 (1978), pp. 247-249.

37. Gerras, *Complete Book of Vitamins.*

38. Carolynn E. Townsend. *Nutrition and Diet Modifications.* Albany, N.Y.: Delmar, 1972, p. 33.

39. Howard and Herbold, *Nutrition in Clinical Care*, p. 114.

40. Benjamin Colimore and Sarah Stewart Colimore. *Nutrition and Your Body*, 2nd edition. Los Angeles, Calif.: Light Wave Press, 1978, p. 20.

41. John Feltman. "Dolomite for the heart," *Prevention* (February 1976), pp. 152-158.

42. Helen W. Lane et al. "Effect of physical activity on human potassium metabolism in a hot and humid environment," *The American Journal of Clinical Nutrition*, 31, 5 (1978), pp. 838-843.

43. Gretchen Mayo Reed. "Confused about potassium? here's a clear, concise guide," *Nursing '74* (March 1974), p. 22.

44. Robert Rodale. "Zinc—how much is not enough?" *Prevention* (September 1976), pp. 23-28.

45. Harold H. Sandstead et al. "Zinc deficiency in pregnant rhesus monkeys: effects on behavior of infants," *The American Journal of Clinical Nutrition* 31, no. 5 (1978), pp. 844-849.

46. Rodale, *Zinc.*

47. Howard and Herbold, *Nutrition in Clinical Care*, pp. 133-134.

48. "Cancer prevention could be right inside your door," *The Body Forum* 2, no. 3 (1977), p. 22.

49. Howard and Herbold. *Nutrition in Clinical Care*, pp. 134-135.

50. C. Edith Weir. *Human Nutrition: Report # 2, Benefits from Nutrition Research*, USDA, 1971.

51. Passwater, *Super-nutrition.* New York: Pocket Books, pp. 93-94.

52. Ibid., p. 95.

53. "What's new? lecithin helps remove tissue cholesterol," *Geriatrics* 33, no. 9 (1978), p. 15.

54. "An apple a day will at least keep the cardiologist away," *Rutgers Alumni Magazine* (December 1977), pp. 26-27.
55. N. Painter. "Diverticular disease of the colon and constipation," *Nursing Times* 68 (1972), pp. 620-621.
56. Joan Jennings. "Bran wards off the 'bane of elders,'" *Prevention* (March 1976), pp. 163, 166-168, 170-176.
57. Sheila and Gerald Bordin. "Bran: roughage that's rough on iron," *New England Journal of Medicine* 294, no. 1 (1976), p. 57.
58. Doris J. Rapp."Is your unusual medical problem an allergy?" *Let's Live* (April, 1976), pp. 96-98.
59. John Diamond. *BK Behavioral Kinesiology.* New York: Harper & Row, 1979, pp. 8-22, 126.
60. D. Mark Hegsted. "The development of a national nutrition policy." *Focus on Health Maintenance and Prevention of Illness.* Wakefield, Mass.: Contemporary Publishing, 1975, pp. 65-71.
61. Howard and Herbold, *Nutrition in Clinical Care*, p. 15.
62. Frances Moore Lappe, *Diet for a Small Planet*, pp. 31-40.
63. "3 drinks linked to hypertension risk," *NIAA Information and Feature Service* (December 21, 1977), p. 2.
64. Ben F. Feingold. "A reply by Dr. Ben Feingold on the Kaiser-Permanente diet," *Behavior Today* (August 8, 1977), pp. 6-7.
65. E. Neige Todheinter and William J. Darby. "Guidelines for maintaining adequate nutrition in old age," *Geriatrics* 33, no. 6 (1978), pp. 49-56.
66. "National awareness of fetal syndrome sought," *NIAAA Information and Feature Service* (September 8, 1977), p. 1.
67. Gerras, *The Complete Book of Vitamins*, pp. 209-210, 230-231, 240, 278.
68. Edward J. Calabrese. *Pollutants and High Risk Groups.* New York: Wiley, 1978, pp. 93-114.
69. Ibid., p. 101.
70. "Radiation poisoning." In *Natural Healing*, ed. by Mark Bricklin. Emmaus, Pa.: Rodale, 1976, pp. 449-452.
71. P. Hernuss, *Strahlentherapie* 150, no. 5 (1975), pp. 500-506.
72. Calabrese, *Pollutants*, p. 181.
73. Harold J. Taub, "Kelp can guard against radiation dangers," *Prevention* (August 1972), pp. 31-49.
74. "Radiation poisoning," in *The Practical Encyclopedia of Natural Healing*, by Mark Bricklin. Emmaus, Pa.: Rodale, 1976, pp. 449-452.
75. Calabrese, *Pollutants*, p. 106.
76. Ibid., pp. 108-109.
77. Ibid., p. 109.
78. Ibid., pp. 112-113.
79. Indra Devi. *Yoga For Americans.* Englewood Cliffs, N.J.: Prentice-Hall, 1959, pp. 172-173.
80. Ardith Blackwell and William Blackwell. "Relieving gas pains," *American Journal of Nursing* 75, no. 1 (1975), pp. 66-67.

81.	Anthony Hartie. "Obesity: environmental control of eating," *Nursing Mirror* 141 (November 1975), pp. 47–49.

82.	Jane Kinderlehrer. *Confessions of a Sneaky Organic Cook . . . Or How to Make Your Family Healthy When They're Not Looking.* New York: Signet, 1972.

83.	Charles E. Butterworth. "The skeleton in the hospital closet," *Nutrition Today* (March/April 1974), pp. 4–8.

3

Being Fit

This chapter focuses on ways in which you can help yourself and others to assess fitness levels and take action to increase your fitness. Continue to remember that fitness is only one part of a wellness approach. Some topics that will be explored are: monitoring your own fitness by checking pulse and blood pressure, through physical and mental health examination, and through health records; methods of natural healing to use with yourself; and types of and benefits from exercise.

MONITORING FITNESS

What do we know about keeping fit? It seems clear that having a large number of laboratory tests done yearly has little relationship to keeping fit. A number of authors [1-14] have examined the use of screening tests and have found strong evidence for regular examinations of only three types: blood pressure, self-examination and physician examination of the breast, and Pap smears.

This does *not* mean that you should not have laboratory tests *if* you have some physical symptom or sign; these could be telling you something is wrong with your body. What it does indicate is that large-scale screening of people, such as the annual physical exam, has failed to enhance wellness. The criteria adopted by the World Health Organization are that it is beneficial to test for the presence of a disease only if:

1. the disease the test detects has a significant effect on the quality and quantity of life;
2. acceptable methods of treatment are available;
3. the disease has a period without symptoms, during which treatment can reduce the disease or death rate;
4. treatment during the period without symptoms yields a better result than would be obtained by delaying treatment until symptoms appear;
5. tests are available at reasonable cost to detect the condition in the period prior to symptoms;
6. the number of occurrences of the illness is large enough to justify the cost of screening.

Figure 3-1 lists detection tests that *have* been demonstrated to enhance wellness by meeting these criteria [2-7]. Figure 3-2 lists tests for which there is *no objective evidence* to support their use [8-14].

Many people think that their physician looks out for their health. In practice, people decide when to go for help, whether to take the advice they are given, what to eat, how much exercise to get, and when and if they will have children. On the other hand, people often seek medical advice for minor complaints such as colds; this is strange because this is a disease that cures itself. And they go to emergency rooms often, but many of those visits are not for emergencies [15]. Finally, although physicians or other health practitioners frequently prescribe drugs or medications, 25 to 50 percent of all clients never take them [16]. Fortunately, most illnesses are self-limiting, and the human body has a miraculous ability to cure itself.

Physicians deal best with serious *illnesses.* You are best at monitoring *health* and *wellness.* However, first you must learn specific ways of monitoring your fitness. Chapter 2, Eating Well, should give you some aid in monitoring your nutritional state.

For a number of diseases, there is a lack either of the ability to make an early diagnosis or of giving effective treatment, or both. Also, most diseases or injuries do not require immediate treatment. With the exception of breathing or major circulation problems, most cases can be handled, at least for a while, by people themselves. Even broken bones do not require immediate care if you know how to care for yourself. (Refer to the Appendix, Wellness Resources, for books and courses that can help you learn how to care for illnesses and injuries, and when to go to a physician for further assistance.)

Although practitioners who order many laboratory tests are considered the most competent in monitoring illness, in reality many laboratory tests often confuse the issue and can in themselves be harmful. This occurs because there is a possibility that the test results may show up an illness when you do not have it, *or* give false negative results leading to an omission in needed treatment [17, 18]. The less serious the illness is, the less likely it is that laboratory tests will help the practitioner make a diagnosis. Also, no laboratory test is 100 percent sensitive—that is, able to detect when a disease is present—*or* 100 percent specific—that is, able to distinguish between those who do have the disease and those who do not. This means that if a test is 95 percent specific, five out of every 100 people given the test will show a *false positive*, that is, as having the disease when they do not! What you need to do in relation to laboratory tests is to ask physicians and other practitioners: How likely is it that I have the disease even if the test should prove positive? Once you receive an answer, you will have to weigh the advantages and disadvantages of having the test, and the chances that you may not have the disease yet may show a positive on your test results. One major consideration in this decision is the potential danger of the test; if the test is not dangerous to you, you may choose to have the test even though you know there is a chance you may seem to have the illness (based on the test results) when you actually do not have it. On the other hand, it is important to weigh the possible disadvantage of thinking you may be ill or handicapped (based on a false positive test result) when you actually do not have the disease. Also, there is the problem of self-fulfilling prophecy. Some people who have been labeled as having illnesses when they do not take on a "sick role" or receive overprotective messages from family members, thus resulting in a psychological disability. This is what was found to happen in children who were diagnosed as having heart murmurs (see Figure 3-2); physically they outgrew their murmurs but psychologically they were handicapped by their diagnosis.

For all these reasons, you need to begin to monitor your own health and wellness, rather than counting solely on medical practitioners. Perhaps the best place to start is by learning how to monitor your pulse and blood pressure.

Monitoring Pulse

Some facts you might want to consider when learning about your pulse rate are:

Pulse is the rate at which your heart beats.

Taking your pulse is not a sign you are looking for illness.

To enhance your wellness, work to make your heart beat more slowly through weight control, diet, and exercise.

The ideal heart rate varies from person to person, increasing somewhat with age.

At rest, your heart should beat about 70 times a minute.

Wait until you feel relaxed, and then place the first two fingers of one hand on the hollow spot on wrist just below the thumb of your opposite hand. Press lightly, trying to feel the blood pulsing through the artery. Take your time, and do not be discouraged if you cannot feel it right away.

Use a watch with a sweep-second hand, and count how many times you feel the pulse in 30 seconds; then multiply by two to derive your pulse rate at rest.

To test your fitness, take your pulse rate before exercise such as 15 minutes of fast walking, jogging, cycling, or swimming. Take your pulse again five minutes after completing the exercise, and again five minutes after that. If you are fit, your pulse should return to its resting rate after ten minutes. If you are extremely fit, it should happen after five minutes [19].

Another point to keep in mind is that rate of pulse is only one aspect to note. The strength of the beat, and whether beats are missed or occurring at regular intervals, are also important. A healthy pulse is slow, strong, and steady.

Monitoring Blood Pressure

The main detection test for heart disease is the annual blood pressure check, as shown in Figure 3-1. Generally, adult blood pressure is considered normal if it falls between 140/90 and 100/60. A reading of 120/80 is considered typical for a healthy adult between the ages of 20 and 39.

Often health care practitioners are most concerned about the lower number, the *diastolic pressure*, or the reading of the heart at rest. (The *systolic pressure*, or upper number, is a measure of the force of the heart when it pumps or beats.) The High Blood Pressure National Task Group has classified groups according to blood pressure and recommended appropriate treatment. These are:

Group 1: From 90 to 105 diastolic pressure. Drugs have not been shown to be helpful for this group, and people in this category should refuse them if ordered, telling physicians, "I'd like to bring down my pressure by natural means, such as exercise, adequate rest, a low-salt diet, no smoking, keeping my cholesterol low by diet, and by learning stress-reduction techniques."

Group 2: Diastolic pressure between 105 and 120. This is classified as moderate hypertension. Diuretics ("water pills") are often prescribed. People who take them should check to see whether the diuretic prescribed promotes the excretion of potassium and magnesium. If it does, they should eat plenty of bananas, oranges, dried peaches and apricots.

Group 3: Diastolic pressure between 120 and 140. Hypertension is classified as severe. Diuretics may be prescribed; note group 2.

Group 4: Diastolic pressure over 140. Hypertension is classified as very severe. Diuretics may be prescribed; note group 2.

For groups 3 and 4, drugs that relax blood vessels may also be combined with diuretics. You should learn to monitor your own blood pressure and use natural means to bring it within normal ranges so you will most likely not have to take medications, since these often have very uncomfortable effects such as nausea, and they may have long-term effects not yet known.

You can be the best monitor of your own blood pressure. Readings taken in doctor's or nurse's offices may be above your actual blood pressure if you are anxious about the visit or have been rushed. For these and other reasons, regular measurements by you are probably the best wellness-enhancing way to proceed.

You can purchase blood pressure equipment from medical

supply houses, pharmacies, or mail-order houses. The entire set usually costs between $20 and $40, and it is well worth the investment. Directions are usually supplied; however, you may find the instructions given in Figure 3-3 of additional assistance. If you are living alone purchase a sphygmomanometer that has a stethoscope head built right into it. Although this device is not quite as accurate, it does make taking blood pressure much easier. If you live with others, you can purchase the standard type of equipment and take one another's blood pressure. Even conventional equipment can be used by one person by clamping the pressure dial to the cuff or propping it up against something stable so readings can be taken. Even the cuff can be placed around one's own arm if it is fastened together while it is still on the table; then the fastened cuff can be slipped up the arm to the proper position, and that arm can rest on a table, palm upward [20, 21].

It is important to remember that children's blood pressure cannot be taken on adult equipment. Separate equipment will have to be purchased for them. With the rise in juvenile hypertension, this, too, is a good investment. In addition, it provides a vehicle for children to be taught how their bodies work.

Physical Examination

The yearly physical. Although it has not been demonstrated that a yearly physical is of any value in preserving health [22], it can be used as a self-detection measure. There are some parts of the physical examination that may prove more useful than other parts; if you wish to know more you can refer to the Appendix, Wellness Resources, pp. 339–360.

Height and weight. You should know the ideal weight for your height, and you should weigh yourself regularly to see how your weight fluctuates. Regular weigh-ins not only alert you to increased and decreased weight due to over- or under-eating, but they can also provide cues about food allergies, depression, and some illnesses.

Temperature. It is important for everyone to know their normal temperature, since the temperature is a signal of the body's attempts to fight off infection or invasion. Although the average normal temperature is 98.6°F, many people have normal temperatures a degree or so above or below that point, and so a low-grade fever for a person who has a normal temperature of 96.6 would be lower than for the person who has a normal temperature of 98.6. Figure 3–4 includes some instruction you could use to take your own or someone else's temperature.

Skin. An examination of the skin can reveal areas of irritation or infection, swelling, pimples, rashes, moles, warts, boils, chancres (sign of first-stage syphilis; a painless ulcer that appears on genitals or mouth or face from 10 to 90 days after sexual contact with an infected person). Some of these clues are, of course, more serious than others. Chancres need immediate medical attention, and moles that change radically should also receive swift care. Swelling could be due to clothing that is too tight, food or drug reactions, poor circulation, too much salt, kidney problems, or poor nutritional status. Where the swelling is and what other symptoms go along with the swelling are what counts. Anyone who has a number of distressing symptoms should be encouraged to seek medical help.

Rashes may be due to a number of causes. Distribution of the rash is often a cluse to its cause. If a woman only has a rash on her face and has just changed cosmetics, she is probably allergic to the cosmetic. Plants such as poison ivy will cause skin irritation in those areas that have been exposed to the oils of the plant either directly through contact or indirectly through scratching. Some people may be allergic to certain synthetic fabrics, or the dyes used therein, and this could be the source of the rash. Examination of the skin can be done during or after a shower or bath. It is important to get to know your body surface and to observe changes and record them. You can also learn to use your skin as a measure of nutritional status. In a well-nourished, healthy young person, the skin quickly returns to the normal shape when released after a fold of it is picked up between thumb and index finger. With age, some of this elasticity is lost, but only the very old should have inelastic, paper-thin skin. Skin is also an indication of overweight. For example, if a fold of skin is pinched under the upper arm or at waist level, the resulting fold should be no thicker than one inch for the female person who is not overweight.

Eyes. The eyes are an important part of the body to examine. Yellowing of the skin and eyes indicates jaundice, a symptom of liver damage; speedy treatment is needed from a doctor or nurse practitioner. Burning, itching, or tearing of the eyes may indicate eyestrain; people with these problems can have their eyes examined, rest their eyes more frequently, and avoid overusing them.

Breasts. Women ought to examine their breasts for lumps after each menstrual period. Figure 3-5 gives directions to use for breast self-examination. Once they begin to practice doing the exam, women learn how *their* breast tissue feels. Any changes in breast tissue, especially lumps, should be immediately reported to a physician.

Lymph nodes. Lymph nodes protect the body by fighting off infection. Nodes can become enlarged as a result of infections—as the body tries to heal itself—or due to problems that require additional assistance. For this reason, you need to be able to examine specific lymph nodes regularly and note changes. Figure 3-6 gives directions for examining lymph nodes in various parts of the body. Size of the node, and any sensitivity or pain noted when examining the node, are important. For example, tiredness, fever, sore throat, painful swollen glands in the neck, armpits, and groin, pain in the upper left-hand side of abdomen, and (perhaps) jaundice are symptoms of infectious mononucleosis. When this group of symptoms occurs together, you should seek health care from a physician or qualified nurse practitioner. Those who learn to examine their own lymph glands need to know that these glands should be flat and often difficult to find *unless* there is a current inflammation *or* unless there was an earlier infection, now cleared up, where nodes can be felt because they have become sites of drainage [23].

Abdomen. You may find it difficult to examine your own abdomen, but you can learn to give instructions for this examination to a trusted friend or family member. Pain or swelling of abdominal organs can be indications of liver, appendix, or spleen problems. Figure 3-7 gives directions for this examination. A healthy abdomen will be soft, and the examiner will feel no organs or masses unless the examinee is very thin. Sometimes it may be possible to feel the edge of the liver, but most of it lies under the ribs in the upper right-hand side of the abdomen. The spleen is located in the upper left-hand side of the abdomen. If it is enlarged, as with mononucleosis, the examiner will be able to feel a firm mass. If there is difficulty with the appendix, the one being examined will feel pain around the navel and will suffer from loss of appetite, nausea, and vomiting. If the appendicitis progresses without action being taken, the examinee will feel tenderness in the right lower section of the abdomen on examination that is made worse by coughing. If this happens medical help should be sought immediately since the appendix is probably blocked by small pieces of feces and will have to be removed, or it will rupture and cause serious infection throughout the body. A white blood cell count can confirm the diagnosis made by examination.

The thyroid. You can learn to examine your thyroid gland by looking and feeling for enlargement. Directions for this examination appear in Figure 3-8. The thyroid gland is not usually visible, unless it is enlarged.

Fitness Record

The first part of Figure 3-9 can be used to assess your physical fitness. The second section of Figure 3-9 is an immunization record. In general, once children have had their basic immunizations, they need few as adults. The only ones recommended by Donald Vickery, M.D., are [24]:

a tetanus booster every ten years unless exposed to a puncture wound; in that case, get a tetanus booster if it has been more than five years since the last booster

a diphtheria booster for those who are at high risk from exposure to the disease, such as hospital workers

There is an unsettled debate about the benefits and negative effects of childhood immunization [25, 26], and you may wish to do further reading on the subject.

Mental Health Examination

Mental health is not merely the absence of disturbing symptoms. Psychiatric diagnosis, such as of schizophrenia, are of no help and can, in fact, be harmful because once people are labeled as having a particular diagnosis, they tend to act and be treated that way whether they originally had the difficulty or not. There are many people working and functioning who show the classical symptoms of this or that psychiatric "illness." Likewise, there are people in psychiatric hospitals who are there primarily because they do not know how to get a job or deal with parents or bosses. Therefore, the question of who has which psychiatric diagnosis is of little value. What *is* of value are some general measures of ability and satisfaction in living. You *can* learn to become *aware* of areas of satisfaction and dissatisfaction, because unrecognized dissatisfaction can lead to anxiety, depression, and other problems.

The other area where you can begin to influence your mental health is by controlling sources of *stress*. It seems quite clear that stress plays a role in the development of physical, mental, and psychosomatic illness. Probably no illness is completely physical or completely mental. The mind influences the body, and vice versa. On the other hand, people cannot simply avoid stress and hope to be healthy. Some stress is normal and expected. In fact, some people thrive on certain types of stress, and what is stressful for one person may not be stressful to another. It is what the person does with the stress that is important. You can learn to detect sources of stress by becoming aware of common situations, such as changes, that are likely to cause it. Most people can take only so many changes over a period of time without developing a physical illness [27].

There are two procedures you can use to help yourself to become more aware of your satisfaction and dissatisfaction with your life. The third section of the Fitness Record, Figure 3-9, can be used for this purpose. Although the section is entitled Mental Health Examination, social, work, and even spiritual aspects are tapped. Figure 3-10 can be used to help evaluate sources of stress.

NATURAL HEALING AND FITNESS

Human beings have been evolving for over three million years on earth. During that time, our bodies have developed ways of protecting and healing themselves. If we get cuts or burns, we do not have to tell our bodies to heal them. Compared to the other complex processes the body is capable of, healing a cut is a simple task. The body knows, for example, how to analyze thousands of substances from the environment and protect itself from harmful ones by creating antibodies to neutralize the harm. There are cells to bring nutrients to other cells, others to break down bacteria, and still others to carry away waste products. Each cell knows what to do without any intervention from us. Our natural healing processes contribute to fitness, but only if we do not interfere with them.

When you are tense, you prevent blood from fully circulating, and it releases abnormal hormonal secretions to damaged areas. Likewise, when you do not keep damaged areas clean, you interfere with normal body processes that heal. You also interfere if you continually bombard your digestive system with too much food or the wrong kind of food. If you unthinkingly take medications or treatments without asking about the positive and negative effects of these substances and procedures, you probably discount your own natural healing ability. Thinking negative thoughts, picturing negative images can also work against your body's natural healing processes. Entertaining ideas of peace, harmony, and love and accepting your feelings of fear, anger, and jealousy as they arise will more likely lead to a body that is relaxed, radiant, alert, and that has a natural flow of blood, energy, and hormones [28].

It will be useful for you to try to find a health care practitioner who views natural healing and fitness as you do. Health care workers who view healing as a natural process also tend to view illness as a symptom of disharmony or stagnation in the entire mind/body. When you think negatively about the health-enhancing aspects of your life—such as nutrition, exercise, medical or health care—you cannot use your own innate healing powers to work with these other aspects.

Health care workers and those who practice a holistic approach think of the mind and body as one inseparable system. In this view, it follows that what people think, believe, and feel is experienced in their bodies. This idea explains why people who are given a *placebo* such as a "sugar pill," and told it will help them, often get better. Hope and trust in a medication or treatment seems to mobilize people to heal themselves. Although many health care practitioners discount the placebo effect as a potent tool in the relationship between client and caregiver, the use of this tool has proved highly effective and certainly has fewer harmful side effects than do many medications.

When health care workers and clients work together to change belief systems about self-healing, some spectacular effects occur [29-36]:

> Some people who have been diagnosed as having incurable cancer and who used relaxation, deep breathing techniques, and visualization have shrunk the cancer or completely rid their bodies of it.

> Clients at the UCLA Pain Control Unit use hypnosis, biofeedback, acupuncture, relaxation exercises, nutritional and family counseling, and dialogue with self to rid themselves of pain.

> People who suffer from migraine headaches can rid themselves of the problem through dialogue with their inner selves.

> Some male clients who have hemophilia are able to control their bleeding through the use of self-hypnosis.

Clients with menstrual cramps use visualization to reduce their discomfort.

Clients who are constipated use visualization to increase their bowel regularity.

Clients with leukemia, glaucoma, learning disabilities, inability to walk after being hit by a truck, chronic backache, diverticulitis, psoriasis, and hepatitis have been taught to use visualization to heal themselves.

Humor and laughter are being used as sources of healing for physical and mental distress.

Clients have been taught to use self-hypnosis to control pain from extensive body burns, back problems, emotional suffering stirred by pain, colitis, weight reduction, phobias, and hair pulling.

Clients have learned to use biofeedback and hypnosis to increase the temperature of their fingers (as a way to decrease migraine headaches).

The above examples are only a sample of the many ways clients have learned to heal themselves. Because the area of self-healing appears to be such a promising one—it is effective, there are no harmful effects, and clients can take responsibility for their own healing without being dependent on external pills, treatments, or helpers—some specifics about some of these techniques will be presented. (Self-hypnosis techniques appear in Chapter 4.)

Visualization

Visualization techniques are based on the idea that what people visualize will come to pass. People who think of a cancer inside them as a horrible, disgusting mass eating them away are using negative imagery. This kind of visualization is apt to end in the client giving in or giving up to the illness. It is a fairly widely accepted theory now that all of us have cancer in some form during our life, but some of us give in to it [37]. Visualization techniques may be one way you can learn to ward off giving in or giving up to illness.

In order to use the visualization technique effectively, you must first be able to put yourself in a receptive, relaxed state. Chapter 4 gives some examples of relaxation exercises that you can use for yourself.

Not everyone is immediately able to use visualization effectively. In fact, some people may complain they are unable to picture the image graphically. This may be due to lack of practice with the visual mode, overdependence on health care practitioners, or a high level of tension. High tension levels can be decreased by increasing the time period used for relaxation exercises, and by making sure to practice in a quiet, comfortable setting that is conducive to relaxation. Sometimes you may still have difficulty vividly seeing images. One thing to do in this case is to examine vivid objects—a lighted candle, a flower, or a bright piece of jewelry—and to look at each object separately, then close your eyes and try to conjure up a mental image of that object. You can repeat the process until you can clearly visualize one or more of the objects. Figure 3-11 gives general directions for using visualization, while Figures 3-12 through 3-15 give directions for specific uses of the visualization technique. You can read the directions slowly, or you can taperecord them and play them when you want to practice visualization.

Current research on the use of this technique documents the relationship between imagery and the course of disease. Dr. Jeanne Achterberg and Dr. Frank Lawlis, two scientists at the University of Texas Health Science Center, are exploring this relationship. So far, they have discovered that the way a particular illness develops and how much rehabilitation can be expected are predictable by the client's images. It seems that clients themselves are able to diagnose and predict the course of their disease. These two scientists are currently using this procedure for people who have cancer, hypertension, and diabetes. Clients are asked to visualize their illness and then to picture their bodies' attempts at healing. Clients who picture their healing white blood cells as ineffective are generally not responding well to medical treatment. Even clients who are unsophisticated and who know little about physiology or medicine are able to use this technique [38].

People who are receiving medications or treatments can learn to visualize these substances and procedures helping them. In this way, they can truly collaborate with health care practitioners. Visualization also seems to have some benefit when carried out by family or friends who are deeply interested in the welfare of the ill person. Visualization exercises are also useful for people who are well and who wish to stay that way [39].

Visualization can even be used to stop the trauma surrounding an accident. In this case, people are asked to repeat their behavior, both in their mental images and in pantomime. People seem to cut off the fear, pain, and anxiety they felt at the time of the accident and unconsciously block their healing powers by cutting off blood flow to the injured part of the body. By reviewing what happened at the time of the injury, including awareness of the injured part, temperature, sounds, words, actions, feelings, attitudes, and thoughts, people can help resume the normal healing process [40]. It is suggested that this kind of approach be used ten seconds after the injury. Since you are unlikely to be around at this time, it is useful to teach your children or other family members how to use this technique so they can use it themselves as a healing measure. Accident-prone people may especially benefit from this knowledge. Visualization techniques are currently being used in collaboration with traditional and medical approaches. They seem to activate the intuitive, wise parts of ourselves and to quiet the rational, logical parts that have not been useful to healing.

Dialogue with Inner Self

Dialogue with Inner Self is a technique used to help people examine the meaning of their illness to them. The dialogue is used to help them to find out what the physical symptoms represent. The dialogue also points the way to release from the symptoms through deciding on a healthier line of action. Dr. Irving Oyle [41] believes that the body often becomes the battleground for ideas and attitudes that conflict with one another. He helps people enter into a dialogue with a mythical figure that he helps them to discover in themselves. He instructs them to go in their mind's eye to a lake and wait for an animal or figure to appear to them. He also tells them that this animal or figure will reveal to them precisely what *they* have been doing to develop the symptom. What this process does is to help people separate themselves from their conflicting feelings or thoughts; it can be valuable to their understanding of where their lives have gone awry. It also builds on the idea that people have intuitive knowledge about themselves, if only they can obtain access to it.

People seem to choose "health advisers" or "inner guides" that reflect what is going on inside of them: those who are cynical often have sarcastic advisers, timid people have timid advisers, and those who do not really want to know what is happening to them choose guides who do not speak.

A main tenet of this theory is that intuitive parts of ourselves are always trying to communicate information to us. Dialogue with Inner Self assists us to gain access to this information. Figure 3-16 gives directions for contacting your health adviser.

Positive Affirmations

Positive affirmations are thoughts people *choose* to think [42]. You may think that thoughts simply occur, yet people *can* learn to think positively as a way of influencing their healing. You can take any positive thought about healing and write it ten to twenty times a day. The thought can be carried with you on a 3 x 5 card, be made into a sign and placed in a prominent spot, or even used as the basis for a needlepoint project. You would need to develop a system so you read or think the affirmation at specified times during the day. Positive affirmations may be especially useful if you are less visually oriented or if you have difficulty with visualization or dialogue with self. Figure 3-17 gives some directions for using positive affirmations.

Yoga

Yoga is a very old method of healing. Its amazing results are now being studied clinically. At Yogic Health Centers in India, records are kept of clients being treated for overweight, diabetes, digestive problems, and breathing problems. In Poland, yoga postures have been found to increase the use of available oxygen by the body. In California, Dr. Barbara Brown has concluded from studying the brain waves of yogis that most illnesses will eventually be treated by establishing healthy brain wave patterns. Dr. Eugene Pendergrass, past president of the American Cancer Society, has stated that cancer is affected by emotional distress and that our minds are capable of inhibiting or aiding the progress of this illness.

Yoga is in tune with a wellness approach. It is based on the concept that a healthy person has a harmonious balance of mind, body, and spirit. More specifically, good health requires a simple, natural diet, exercise in fresh air, a serene, untroubled mind, and a oneness with a higher being or order. Yoga postures are meant to normalize the functions of the body by regulating breathing, circulation, digestion, and metabolic processes. Also, glands, organs, and the nervous system are stimulated and relaxed. The way this is achieved is through placing the body in various postures while using deep-breathing techniques. Each exercise creates a different relationship between the body and the force of gravity. Thus, some postures open up the chest and lung cavity and increase breathing capacity, others stretch, tone, and lubricate the spinal cord or joints, bring blood and nutrients to the brain or extremities, or take the pressure off internal organs. Yoga exercises seem to assist the healing process by removing impurities and obstructions. By gradually stretching and strengthening the body, clients can also achieve inner peace and respect for themselves.

The following are some of the ways in which yoga has been used in healing:

The yoga respiration is used to prevent pneumonia in people who overdose in suicide attempts.

Children who have asthma learn to strengthen their lungs by using the yoga Complete Breath (a nurse puts a plastic duck on their abdomen and tells them to watch the duck "float up and down on the tummy waves").

People practice the Complete Breath, the Knee to Chest position, Sun Salutation, Shoulder Stand, and Corpse Pose to obtain healing sleep when they are distraught.

Those with emphysema (a lung disease) use the Complete Breath Locust, Grip, and Shoulder Stand while visualizing healing circulation occurring in their lungs.

Women with menstrual disorders seem to benefit from the Shoulder Stand, Plow, Fish, Uddiyana, Cobra, and Posterior Stretch.

Those who have a cold practice the Lion and Shoulder Stand to soothe throat and sinus congestion and drain secretions.

Those with varicose veins increase cirulation to their legs by practicing the Shoulder Stand.

Men with prostate difficulties and people with constipation practice the Kneeling Pose.

People who suffer from rheumatism practice the Mountain, Shoulder Stand, Twist, Knee to Chest position, and Posterior Stretch, while visualizing the cleansing of waste material from their joints.

Those with backaches practice the Corpse Pose, Locust, Plow, and Knee to Chest position while visualizing healing blood nourishing and healing their back muscles [43].

Yoga postures are meant to be done when the stomach is empty. You should choose a well-ventilated, quiet room. A rug or pad should be used, and loose-fitting clothes must be worn. Generally, a backward-bending posture is balanced by a forward-bending position. Postures should be performed slowly, in a meditative mood.

Never force, strain, or bounce to achieve a pose. Each person takes the pose to his or her maximum stretch; no pain should ever be felt. Directions for some of the more simple and basic postures appear in Figures 3-18 through 3-21 [44, 45]. Other poses can be found in Yoga texts; some of these are described in the Appendix. Beginners can have the directions for the poses read to them until they are familiar with what to do, or they can taperecord the directions and play them back.

Thump Your Thymus

Dr. John Diamond believes that illness is due to energy imbalance [46]. Using this theory, it is easy to assume that if we can become aware of energy imbalances when they first occur, we will be preventing illness. Most prevention of illness is now practiced at the secondary level: for example, people who have had a heart attack want to know how to prevent another one from occurring. If early energy imbalances can be detected, perhaps there will be fewer chronic illnesses.

Dr. Diamond reports that he has never seen a client with a chronic degenerative disease who did not have an underactive thymus gland [47]. Because of his extensive research, he has concluded that the thymus gland is the clue to energy balance in the body. He has found that it is the first organ to be affected by stress. If your thymus tests weak (see test in Chapter 2, p. 32), you can reactivate and re-energize it by "thumping."

To locate the thymus, place the fingertips on the skin at the point where the second rib joins the breastbone (the sterno-mandibular joint) [48]. This is about three inches below the collarbone, in the middle of the chest. Dr. Diamond suggests that you learn to tap your thymus gently ten or twelve times a day as a preventive measure [49]. This will activate the thymus and keep your energy level balanced. Thymus thumping also seems useful for people who are already ill and who need increased muscular strength or energy flow.

Laying on of Hands

Laying on of hands is one of the oldest and most widely used methods of healing. People use this method when they physically comfort a child or hold a loved one. Touch provides energy, reassurance, and a transfer of energy or strength. Although energy itself is neutral, mental health counselors and others who are open to clients' problems have been known to report feeling depressed after seeing a depressed client; the client, on the other hand, looks and feels better! What seems to have happened here is a transfer of energy. Nurses, physicians, physical therapists, parents, and others who may frequently be called upon to use physical touch or energy transfer may require laying on of hands themselves. Chellis Glendinning [50] suggests several forms of protection and cleansing to strengthen those who strengthen others: meditation imagining a white light surrounding yourself, or channeling energy through your feet through the floor while working or "healing," or taking a walk or airing the room after the experience is over. Dolores Krieger, a doctorally prepared nurse who uses therapeutic touch, has recently been studying the relaxing effects of touch [51-52].

Laying on of hands can be practiced when an imbalance has already manifested itself as a physical problem; it can also be used as a way of removing energy blockages or an imbalance for which there are no distressing symptoms as yet [53].

Figures 3-22 and 3-23 give some directions for laying on of hands.

EXERCISE

Forty-five percent of Americans *never* exercise. This is especially frightening because inactivity has been linked to hypertension, chronic fatigue, physiological inefficiency, premature aging, poor musculature, inadequate flexibility, lower-back pain, injury, tension, obesity, arteriosclerosis, and coronary heart disease [54].

Although the effects of inactivity are startling, the benefits of keeping fit through exercise are just as amazing. The benefits of exercise include: an increased ability to manage stress; greater self-confidence; decreased depression; better eating habits; decreased smoking; better ability to sleep; less use of stimulants, decreased use of alcoholic drinks, better weight control; better ability to relate to other people; lowered heart rate; decreased blood pressure, less body fat; decreased blood cholesterol; increased air flow through nasal passages; reduced joint stiffness; better support for the skeletal structure; increased circulation to heart, arteries, lungs, and all body cells; help for those with diabetes and glaucoma; more positive work attitude; improved work performance; decreased tension; and fewer injuries [55–57].

There is some controversy about what types of exercise are best, but there is generally agreement about the following:

> Jogging is the most efficient and inexpensive approach to enhancing endurance and increasing cardiovascular fitness. Since running fast is not of particular advantage, jogging can be begun in stages by people of *all ages* and even by those who have been ill and require rehabilitation [58].

> Bicycling contributes to fitness of the heart, and it can be done at any age, alone or in company. However, it can cause some cerebral imbalance and requires thymus thumping to restore balance [59].

> Swimming is total body conditioning that is particularly good for clients recovering from hip, knee, and ankle problems. It neglects the weight-bearing, antigravity musculature of the body; perhaps it should be combined with vigorous exercises that do provide a maximum of exercise in a minimum amount of time.

> Cross-country skiing is excellent for fitness.

> Walking is excellent for reconditioning (after illness) and conditioning if done at a brisk, steady pace. It can be done at any age, anywhere, alone or with others; it requires no equipment or money [60]. It also enhances brain balance [61].

Questions You Might Ask about Exercise

What can I do to get rid of my pot belly?

A pot belly is usually due to lack of tone in your abdominal muscles. The best exercise is doing situps. These should be done with knees bent and arms at sides, so as not to put undue strain on the back.

Will sauna belts or rubber suits help me to lose weight?

No. All you will lose is water and minerals; when you drink fluids, you will gain back any weight you lost. And if you lose a lot of minerals from perspiring, you might even be worse off unless you replace them too.

Can I lose weight by walking?

Yes. If you walk for one-half hour a day for a year, you will lose nearly 20 pounds while eating the same amount as you did prior to beginning your exercise program.

What is the best kind of exercise to do if I only have 15 minutes a day?

Walking is probably the bext exercise, since you do not have sufficient time to do warm-up and cool-down exercises. You might want to consider why you only allow yourself 15 minutes a day. Is your health only worth 15 minutes? Can you change your life style, get up earlier, use your lunch hour or break to walk, or arrange your time better? You might be better off taking a walk in the evening rather than watching television. That way, you will not be so tempted to snack.

Won't exercise increase my appetite?

Food may taste better to you after exercise, but vigorous exercise tends to normalize, not increase, the appetite. Your thirst *may* increase with exercise. It is wise not to drink soft drinks, since these add extra calories, or—in the case of diet sodas—contain harmful sweeteners. Water is the most refreshing and thirst-quenching drink [62].

What is the minimal amount I have to exercise to be fit?

Fitness seems to depend on engaging in sustained exercise that mildly stresses the heart and lungs. Stop-and-go exercise, such as tennis, usually end in less fitness than ongoing pursuits such as jogging, walking, and swimming. Yoga may also be thought of as a conditioning type of exercise when done by the serious student. However, it is possible to do one or two yoga postures in a half-hearted way. In this case, little conditioning effect can hope to be achieved, although clients may gain additional benefits, such as increased circulation. Certainly the yogis of India who were able to control their heart and breathing rates were fit, but few Americans are that diligent in their practice.

Daily exercise is best, but three or four sessions a week may keep you fit. It is probably better to do 30 minutes of exercise three times a week than 90 minutes once a week. In general, fitness means endurance, not strength or speed. To build and maintain endurance, regular exercise is needed. There are three kinds of fitness to be aware of: muscular, skeletal (flexibility), and cardiovascular (strength and health of the heart and blood vessels) [63]. Exercise that makes you fit in all three areas is the best. So, clients who only jog ought also to do some yoga and 10 minutes of rope jumping to build up flexibility and to condition the upper part of the body. Calisthenics are not generally recommended, since they are not smooth and tend to lead to injuries unless done under careful supervision.

How can I tell if I'm increasing my fitness?

By taking your pulse before, during, and after your exercise on a regular basis, you can begin to see a reduced rate with increasing exercise if you are increasing your fitness. Adults usually have a resting heart rate of about 60 to 80 beats per minute. Raising the heart rate to 120 beats per minute and sustaining it for fifteen minutes is usually sufficient for fitness to occur. Other signs that you are increasing your fitness are that you feel your heart pumping hard when building endurance, your body begins to feel more alive as there is more warmth and a free flow of oxygen in your tissues, and your pulse returns to its resting rate more and more quickly after you stop exercising [64, 65].

If I exercise too much, will I hurt myself?

Both amount and intensity of exercise can be harmful if your body is not ready for it. For that reason, it is best to start off any exercise program with some warm-ups that slowly awaken the body, to plan a program of exercise that *slowly* builds up to increasing fitness, and always to end an exercise period with a cooling-down period, including stretching exercises (see Figure 3-24). Figure 3-25 shows a sample exercise program for a woman who is 45 years old. If you are worried about stressing yourself too much, you can calculate the rate your pulse should be for your age so you will not overexert yourself. I will show you how to do it using my age and resting pulse rate [66]:

Subtract *your age* from the standard maximum heart rate possible, for example:

$$\begin{array}{r} 220 \\ -38 \ \text{(age)} \\ \hline 182 \ \text{(maximum attainable} \\ \text{heart rate)} \end{array}$$

Subtract your resting heart rate: $\quad -56$

to find a subtotal: $\qquad$ 126 $\qquad\qquad$ 126

Multiply the subtotal by 60 percent: $\qquad$ 0.60 and by 80 percent: $\quad$ 0.80

$\qquad\qquad\qquad\qquad$ 75.60 $\qquad\qquad\qquad$ 100.80

Add your resting heart rate to each: $\qquad$ 56.00 $\qquad\qquad\qquad$ 56.00

$\qquad\qquad\qquad\qquad$ 131.60 $\qquad$ and $\quad$ 156.80

These two pulse rates, 132 and 157, provide the range within which I need to be working in order to achieve a conditioning effect. By taking my pulse as I exercise, I can be sure not to overexert myself. If you insert your age and resting pulse rate, you can calculate your own pulse range for exercise.

Do I need to have an electrocardiograph (a stress test) before I start exercising?

Some authorities claim it is useful. Vickery [67] (a physician himself) claims that cardiologists have invented this need, because "There are more cardiologists than are needed" and because stress testing is profitable. Vickery states that there are several reasons why a stress test is unnecessary: First, the stress test itself has a greater risk of giving you a heart attack (a risk level of 30 to 60 percent) than does unaccustomed, severe exercise (a risk level of 6 to 12). So if people develop an exercise program that *gradually* builds them up to a conditioning level, they should have *less than* one-fifth the risk of a heart attack than if they have a stress test. Second, the stress test is not very good at identifying clients who are at high risk for heart attack. (In a study of persons without symptoms of heart disease, 47 percent who tested "abnormal" on the stress test did *not* have heart disease; in another study, 62 percent of those who *did* have heart disease tested "normal" on the stress test [68].) With so little accuracy, a stress test can hardly seem worth the risk the test itself brings.

You can, however, determine whether you need medical supervision to begin exercise. If you answer "yes" to one or more of the following questions and are over 35 years old, you should see your doctor; if you are under 35, only *call* your doctor and tell him or her the exercise program you plan to follow [69]:

Do you have any chest pain when you exert yourself?

Do you get short of breath with mild exertion?

Do you have pain in your legs when you walk but not when you rest?

Do your ankles swell regularly (at times other than when you are menstruating)?

Has a doctor ever told you you have heart disease?

I know I should exercise, but I find it very hard to get started; can you help me?

I have some ideas that may help you. Try to make physical fitness a part of your life by building it into your social life, by saving to buy equipment or clothes that go with the sport or program, by joining a club that participates in the kind of exercise you like, by subscribing to a magazine or borrowing a book on the topic. Do some deep thinking about what kind of exercise is right for you. Set reasonable expectations for yourself. Even a little regular exercise will show benefits. If you try to overdo, you will become discouraged. Write a contract, stating your goals for increasing exercise over the next three to six months; have it cosigned by a supportive friend who will not nag you, but who will encourage you to meet your contract. Try to get at least some of your exercise outdoors in a pleasant setting, where you can also enjoy some spiritual renewal.

You might try exercising to music. Bending, stretching, and continuous controlled movement to music is a pleasant way of beginning to get fit. Very young children also like to exercise to music. Preschoolers can be asked to crouch like a frog or kangaroo, to jump around to the music, or to arch like a cat, prance like a pony, hump like a rhinoceros, walk like an elephant, and so on. In fact, even adults can do these kinds of animal movements as a way of strengthening muscles and bones.

I have a mother who is 64; can she exercise?

Yes. People of all ages can exercise. Walking is an excellent exercise; so is yoga. Figure 3–26 gives some exercises that have been developed with the older adult in mind. They are especially useful for offsetting the effects of premature aging. As they are yogic in nature, they are meant to be performed slowly and mindfully. There should be no jerking, pushing, or bouncing. Your mother should strive for a controlled stretch. If your mother is taking medication, has high blood pressure, a chronic spine difficulty, or any other condition that might be irritated, or if she drinks heavily [70, 71], she should check with her health care practitioner or doctor prior to beginning the program. If she decides to go ahead with the exercises, ask her to read the directions found in the section entitled, Yoga.

I'm on bedrest for several weeks; are there any exercises I can do to feel better?

If you have not had major surgery, you can probably do the Complete Breath (Figure 3-19), and you can alternately contract and relax all the muscles of your body. You may be able to rotate your wrists and ankles in circles in both directions, or do other exercises. Be sure to check with your doctor before you do them. If you are able to sit up, you can do the following exercises. Roll your shoulders up to your ears and back down again. Roll your head around from one shoulder to your chest back around to your other shoulder. Bend your toes toward your head; hold; then point your toes away from your body. Bend your knees while lying flat in the bed and hunch your shoulders forward, then press the small of your back into the bed; hold, then release.

Here are some other exercises you can do to improve your posture and circulation:

1. Lie on your back, inhale deeply, and press down with both elbows. Exhale, and relax your elbows.
2. Lie on your stomach, inhale deeply, and turn your head to one side. Press your head down, exhale, and relax. Turn your head to the opposite side and repeat. Rest, and feel the benefits.

If you are in the hospital, let doctor and nurse know you want to do some exercise to keep fit; ask them to help you devise a safe exercise program. Some of the exercises that appear in Chapter 4 may also be useful for you. In addition, exercises like the Cobra Posture (Figure 3-18) can be modified for your use.

Figure 3-1 Detection Tests and Preventive Measures for Major Illnesses [2–7]

Illness	Detection tests	Preventive measures
Heart disease	blood pressure checked at least once per year	have a throat culture when you have a *very* painful sore throat that lasts longer than a few days; if culture is positive, take antibiotic to reduce chance of rheumatic heart disease
	have infants age 1–6 months examined for heart malformations	stop smoking
		exercise
		lose weight or maintain ideal weight
		cut down on fat, sugar, and highly processed foods
Cancer	self-examination of breasts by women	do not get an x-ray without questioning why it is necessary; refuse those that seem unnecessary
	self-examination of the thyroid (for women over 18 years of age who are sexually active) obtain a Pap smear yearly until 2 negative results are obtained, then obtain smears every 3 years to age 35 and every 5 years from age 35–60	stop smoking and being near smokers
		do not participate in sexual activity at an early age and/or with many different partners
	examination of the skin for changes—for example, increase in size, number, or look of moles	know environmental chemicals that are cancer-producing, and work to eliminate them and your exposure to them
	self-examination of the testicles by men	limit drinking alcohol

Figure 3-1 (continued)

Illness	Detection tests	Preventive measures
Cancer (cont.)		limit exposure to the sun and/or use PABA cream to block exposure increase fiber intake try to eat foods not sprayed with dangerous pesticides
Stroke	none, except some strokes are preceded by temporary clumsiness and numbness in hand or foot, temporary blindness in one eye, or slurring of speech: these should be immediately brought to the attention of a physician	same as for heart disease
Diabetes	self-test for sugar in the urine, using Tes-Tape, Clinistix, Clinitest Tabs, Diastix, or similar products available in pharmacies; especially useful for juveniles who have extreme thirst, frequent urination, and weight loss	lose weight increase exercise eat proper diet to date it is not known that anything can be done to prevent juvenile diabetes
Tuberculosis	PPD or Tine Skin Test every year or two for ten years after exposure to tuberculosis	avoid exposure to people who have it

Arthritis	none, except for ankylosing spondylitis; in this case, you should check with a physician if you answer yes to four or five of the following: Have you had back pain for three months or more? Has your back been stiff in the morning? Did the problem start before you were 40? Did the pain and stiffness begin slowly? Does the problem improve with exercise?	some experts think taking dolomite (calcium and magnesium) will ward off osteoarthritis
Gout	possibly uric acid blood test in middle-aged, overweight men with a family history of gout	control weight avoid alcoholic drinks
Venereal disease (VD)	having a culture made from the cervix (opening) to the uterus or penis is useful only for people who have large numbers of sexual partners having a blood test (VDRL, FTA) one to three months after exposure	avoid contact with infected persons use condoms use discretion in choice of sexual partner
Glaucoma	having the eye pressure measures with an instrument called a Schiotz Tonometer once every four years after the age of 40, or once a year after age 30 if anyone in your family has glaucoma	
Anemia	an occasional microhematocrit (not a complete blood count) is reasonable for *children* especially if they are *not* eating an adequate diet	a balanced diet that includes vitamins and iron

Figure 3-1 (continued)

Illness	Detection tests	Preventive measures
Thyroid problems	self-examination for small lump to the side of the Adam's apple those who *have* had radiation treatments for acne or ringworm to the head or neck or for enlarged tonsils or adenoids should have their thyroid examined yearly and learn to do a self-examination of the thyroid	refuse x-rays to the head or neck for acne, ringworm, enlarged tonsils, or adenoids
Mental retardation	if you are pregnant and know of a genetic disease that causes mental retardation in your family, see a genetic counselor, think about getting amniocentesis (test of fluid from uterus or womb); likewise, if you are over 40 if there is phenylketonuria (PKU) in your family, have your baby tested immediately after birth and start him or her on the special PKU diet	if there is genetic illness in your family, get genetic counseling prior to marriage
Kidney disease	urine test for pregnant women	

Figure 3-2 /// 105

Figure 3-2   Questionable Screening Procedures [8-14]

---

1. rectal exams

2. xeromammography (x-ray) of the breast (unless you are over age 40 and your sister or mother has breast cancer)

3. proctosigmoidoscopy (looking into the rectum and lower bowel through a tube) prior to age 50

4. x-ray to detect lung cancer

5. test for hidden blood in the stool prior to age 40

6. glucose tolerance test if elderly (77 to 100 percent will test positive for diabetes when they may not have the illness)

7. coronary arteriograms (they are very complex and have a significant chance of causing disability or death)

8. electrocardiograph stress tests (findings are inconclusive unless you have symptoms of heart disease; the test itself may be disabling)

9. screening for heart murmurs in children (the vast majority of murmurs do not indicate disease; children and parents' reactions may cause them to act *as if* there is a disease when there is not)

10. screening for high levels of uric acid for gout (unless you are a middle-aged, overweight man, with a family history of gout)

11. tests to determine whether you have a high cholesterol level (there is no definitive study to show that lowering the cholesterol level will prevent atherosclerosis or coronary heart disease)

12. tests to determine abnormalities through such procedures as chest x-rays, rectal, gastrophy, urine and sputum cytology

13. x-ray examinations to evaluate lower-back pain

14. tests to identify carriers of sickle cell anemia

15. abdominal x-ray to judge liver size or gastrointestinal bleeding

16. x-ray to detect ankle sprain

17. routine barium enemas for hernia

18. urograms and arteriograms for people with high blood pressure

19. daily (portable) x-rays of all patients in coronary care units (CCUs)

20. bone survey x-rays of people with hyperparathyroidism

21. preemployment x-rays of the chest and spine

22. use of CAT scanner in inappropriate situations

23. any x-rays during pregnancy

Figure 3-3   Teaching Yourself to Take Blood Pressure

Step 1:   Become familiar with the equipment

1.   Look at the sphygmomanometer: It is an inflatable rectangular bag
      (called a cuff) that wraps around your upper arm. A bulb is attached;
      you squeeze this while holding it in your hand, and the cuff inflates.
      Attached to the cuff is a dial with each mark equal to two millimeters or
      points; from this you read your two blood pressures as you deflate the
      cuff, using the valve located above the bulb. Practice opening and closing
      the valve until you get a feel for it.

2.   Look at the stethoscope. It has buttons to place in both ears and tubes
      that lead from the ear buttons down to the instrument's head. This disc
      or head is placed on the arm and is used to magnify sounds.

3.   If you like, while practicing, have another person read the following
      directions.

Step 2:   Getting ready to take the blood pressure

1.   Sit beside a table or platform that is about level with your heart when
      you sit. If the table is too low, use a box or a couple of books to provide
      a surface at the correct level.

2.   Be sure you have not eaten, smoked, or exerted yourself in the past
      half-hour. When taking regular readings, take them at a particular time(s),
      and eliminate other factors that might affect readings; for example, make
      an effort to relax, empty your bladder by going to the bathroom, and
      make sure you are warm enough.

3.   Roll up one sleeve to the shoulder, or remove clothing that covers the
      upper arm.

4.   Deflate the cuff by opening the valve and forcing any air out.

5.   Wrap the cuff around the upper arm above where the arm bends.
      There are self-adhesive surfaces so one end will stick to the other. The cuff
      should be snug, but not binding. The tightness will occur when the cuff
      is inflated.

6.   Put the stethoscope buttons into your ears. Place the instrument's head or
      disc just below where the arm bends, a little toward the inside of the arm.
      If you like, remove the disc and feel that spot with the index finger of
      your hand; you should feel a slight pulse from the artery that is there. Re-
      place the disc over that spot.

Figure 3-3 /// 107

7. Be sure the stethoscope does not touch the cuff or any of its tubes.

8. Make certain that the gauge or dial of the cuff is situated so you can easily read it.

9. Sit back for a few seconds and listen to the cracklings and rumblings you hear. Become accustomed to them so you will not confuse these with the beat of the blood pressure later on.

Step 3:   Inflate the cuff

1. Straighten out the arm wearing the cuff.

2. Let the straight arm rest on the table, platform, box, or books.

3. Relax your arms.

4. Close the valve of the pump, and inflate the cuff rapidly until the gauge reads 160.

5. *Immediately* open the valve and release the pressure, watching the dial, so the pressure moves down 2 to 4 mm a second. Do not keep tight pressure on the arm for longer than a second or two without beginning to release pressure.

Step 4:   Read the blood pressure

1. Listen for the first pulse sounds (like a drumbeat or tap) at between 150 and 110 on the dial; this is the systolic reading, the first pulse sound.

2. Continue to let air out of the cuff, watch the dial, and listen for the end of the pulse sounds at 100 and 60. For a person 45 years old or older, the two pressures may be higher. Sometimes the (seeming) last beat will be followed several points on the gauge later by another beat; count this last beat as the diastolic, then quickly deflate the cuff the rest of the way and remove the cuff. Let the arm rest for at least three minutes prior to taking another reading.

Step 5:   Record the readings

1. Record the upper reading (systolic pressure): for example, 130.

2. Record the lower reading (diastolic pressure): for example, 94, as 130/94.

Figure 3-4   Taking a Temperature with an Oral Thermometer

Step 1:   Preparing the thermometer

1.   Clean the thermometer with cool soapy water or with rubbing alcohol and a cotton sponge. Use friction by rubbing the cotton sponge firmly along the thermometer.

2.   Shake the thermometer down by briskly snapping your wrist up and down three or four times.

3.   Look at the thermometer to make sure it is at 96° or less. You may find it difficult to read the thermometer, because the color of the mercury inside is very like the color of the reflection from the glass. Roll the thermometer back and forth, away from and then toward you, slowly a couple of times until you see a thin line of mercury rising above the silver tip.

Step 2:   Inserting the thermometer

1.   Using an oral thermometer, place the silver-tipped end, and about one-half of thermometer, under the tongue. (*Do not* use a rectal thermometer in the mouth or an oral thermometer in the rectum.)

2.   Leave the thermometer in place for two to three minutes.

Step 3:   Reading the thermometer

1.   Remove the thermometer gently.

2.   Look for the highest mark to which the mercury rises.

3.   Record the reading.

4.   Clean thermometer and put in a safe place in clean container.

Figure 3-5 /// 109

Figure 3-5   Directions for Breast Self-Examination

---

1. Examine your breasts by looking in the mirror at them. First, place your arms at your sides, then place both your arms over your head. The breasts should look about the same, although many women have one breast that is a little larger than the other. Look especially for dimpling of the skin, bulges in one breast, or any *change* in size or shape.

2. Examine your breasts while lying flat. Examine each breast with the hand from the opposite side of the body. Press the breast tissue gently against the chest wall, using the inner fingertips. Roll the tissue between your fingers and the chest wall, moving your fingers in a circular massage motion. Do not pinch the tissue, because all breast tissue feels lumpy then. Examine the inner half of each breast while holding the same-side arm over the head. Examine the outer portion of each breast while holding the same-side arm down at your side. Examine underneath the nipples and over to and including the armpit.

Figure 3-6   Directions for Examining Some of the Lymph Nodes

---

Neck glands

1.   Relax jaw and neck muscles.

2.   Place the first three fingers of each hand immediately below the ears, and move the fingers in a smooth circular motion.

3.   Move the fingers down a short distance and a little to the side, and repeat the circular motion.

4.   Continue moving the fingers down and toward the front of the jaw little by little, until the fingers of one hand are very close to the fingers of the other hand.

5.   Note enlarged glands.

Underarm glands

1.   Drop one arm to the side and relax it.

2.   Use the opposite arm to feel for gland under the arm, with the thumb on the chest and the fingers using a circular movement under the arm, including high into the underarm region.

3.   Note enlarged glands.

Groin glands

1.   Place fingertips in the groin area, and move the fingertips from side to side, using firm pressure.

2.   Move fingertips downward toward the thigh.

3.   Note any enlargement.

Figure 3-7 /// *111*

Figure 3-7   Directions for Examining the Abdomen of Another Person

---

1. Make sure the room temperature is warm enough.

2. Ask the other person to lie on his or her back on a firm surface such as a mat on the floor.

3. Have the person remove any clothing that covers the area from their chest to the hair line of their pelvis, and to place both arms comfortably at the sides of the body or at the back of the head.

4. Ask the other person to bend his or her knees slightly, to take a few deep breaths, and to concentrate on relaxing the abdominal area.

5. Place one hand on top of the other, both palms down, and fingertips touching. Use the top hand to provide pressure, and the bottom hand to feel the abdomen.

6. Move your hands over the entire abdomen, pressing lightly. Ask the other person to signal whenever pain is felt.

7. Note when the person tenses up when you examine an area and ask, "What did you feel?"

8. If the other person complains of being tickled, use slightly firmer pressure.

9. Note and record any areas of tenderness or areas that are rigid to the touch.

Figure 3-8   Directions for Two Methods of Examining the Thyroid Gland

---

Examining the thyroid gland through touch

1.   Feel for the band of cartilage (soft, bonelike material) running down the middle of your throat.

2.   Place the thumb of the right hand on the right-hand side of the cartilage and the three fingers of the right hand on the other side, about 2 inches below the chin.

3.   Swallow, and feel the connection between the two parts of the thyroid as it glides beneath your fingertips. When this happens, you are in the correct place to feel for your thyroid gland. If you do not feel the gliding action, the fingers can be moved up or down slightly and you can swallow again.

4.   Once the correct spot is found, keep the three fingers where they are and move the left hand and place the three fingers of that hand on the same level as the other hand, but slightly to the side of the throat.

5.   Then the fingers of the right hand move around slowly in a circular motion, searching for the thyroid.

6.   The same process is repeated (with the hands reversed) for the right half of the thyroid.

Examining the thyroid gland through inspection

1.   Look in the mirror, searching for any sign of enlargement on either side of the cartilage.

2.   Elevate your chin and look in a small hand mirror for any enlargement while swallowing.

Figure 3-9 /// 113

Figure 3-9   Fitness Record

Directions

Monitor and add data as often as suggested in the text, or if there are symptoms suggesting the need for more examination.

PHYSICAL EXAMINATION

My blood pressure at rest is: My *height* is:

My *pulse* at rest is: My *weight* is:

My normal *temperature* is:

From observing my *skin*, I noticed the following:

From observing my *eyes*, I noticed the following:

From examining my *lymph nodes*, I found:

From examining my *breasts* (woman)—*testicles* (man)—I noticed:

My *abdominal* area is:

RECORD OF IMMUNIZATIONS

I have had the following basic immunizations:

yes   no

.... DPT (diphtheria, pertussis, tetanus) and oral polio virus

.... measles

.... rubella (only for females whose blood test shows no immunity
to rubella)

I have had the following boosters:

yes   no

.... diphtheria dates:

.... tetanus   dates:

(continued)

Figure 3–9 (continued)

ADDITIONAL INFORMATION

Age 7–11 (with symptoms of extreme thirst, frequent urination, and weight loss):

I test my urine for sugar regularly and find:

Sexually Active:

I use the following method of birth control:

I protect myself from VD by:

Those who have been exposed to tuberculosis:

I had a PPD or Tine Test most recently on: (date)

Those who are over 40 or over 30 and have a family history of glaucoma:

I had a Schiotz tonometer test done on: (date)

Those who have a history of genetic disease or who are over 40 and thinking of becoming pregnant:

I plan to tackle the problem of genetic difficulties by completing the following actions:

EXPOSURES TO HARMFUL SITUATIONS

I was exposed to the following illnesses:

1.   date:

2.   date:

3.   date:

I had x-rays of the following kinds:

1.   date:

Figure 3-9 /// 115

2.   date:

3.   date:

I was exposed to the following other situations:

1.   date:

2.   date:

3.   date:

MENTAL HEALTH EXAMINATION

Check *Yes, No,* or *S* (*Somewhat* or *Sometimes*) for each statement

		Yes	No	S
1.	I think I handle stress pretty well at work (school)	......	.....	......
2.	I like my coworkers (peers)	......	.....	......
3.	I think I handle stress pretty well at home	......	.....	......
4.	I get out of the house enough to "do my own thing"	......	.....	......
5.	I seem to share a great deal with my family, and I look forward to being with them	......	.....	......
6.	I have the right numbers (for me) of close friends I share things with	......	.....	......
7.	I feel comfortable in social situations	......	.....	......
8.	I seem to have enough energy to do the things I want to do	......	.....	......
9.	I usually get along pretty well with people	......	.....	......
10.	I get enough respect from others for work I do	......	.....	......
11.	I am able to fully utilize those activities for which I have been trained	......	.....	......
12.	I live pretty comfortably	......	.....	......

(continued)

Figure 3-9 (continued)

		Yes	No	S
13.	I seem to be financially secure	......	.....	......
14.	I feel at ease about spending money	......	.....	......
15.	I participate in activities that give me a boost	......	.....	......
16.	There are people or organizations I can turn to in times of trouble	......	.....	......
17.	I know my strengths	......	.....	......
18.	I know my weaknesses or limitations	......	.....	......
19.	I am willing to take reasonable risks to get what I want	......	.....	......
20.	I feel good about persevering and working toward a goal, even if I don't always get what I want	......	.....	......
21.	I structure my day so I am satisfied with its outcome	......	.....	......
22.	I have some long-term goals, and I am working toward them	......	.....	......
23.	I can change my routine once in a while, without undue discomfort	......	.....	......
24.	I try continually to learn or do new things	......	.....	......
25.	I see illness as part of the challenge of living	......	.....	......
26.	I believe that I can help to cure myself when I am ill	......	.....	......
27.	I believe I have some choice in what happens to me	......	.....	......
28.	If I were going to die this evening, I would not change my life	......	.....	......
29.	I have spent my life choosing what I do, not only in being swayed by peers, bosses, teachers, family, friends, or health care workers	......	.....	......
30.	I have confidence in my future	......	.....	......
31.	My life spreads around me, a series of connected experiences	......	.....	......
32.	I believe there is a reason for my being here	......	.....	......

Figure 3-10 /// 117

Figure 3-10   Changes that May Affect You

Directions:

Below is a list of events that may have happened to you in the past year or may
have affected you. For example, if your husband has trouble with his parents,
it may affect you, too. Rate those events that you think have significance for
you. Rate an event as significant if it changed your usual pattern of activities.
Events may be significant positively—changed your life for the better—or
significant negatively—changed your life for the worse. Those events that you
think change your life a lot negatively are the ones that may be affecting your
health negatively.

	YOUR REACTION				
	Negative		*No*	*Positive*	
	A little	*A lot*	*reaction*	*A little*	*A lot*

SCHOOL

1. started a new school experience ....
2. failed an important exam ....
3. failed a course ....
4. flunked out of school ....
5. dropped out of school ....
6. graduated from school ....

other school experiences that had an impact on me

7.

8.

WORK

1. started a new job or business ....
2. trouble with boss ....

(continued)

Figure 3–10 (continued)

		Negative		No	Positive	
		A little	*A lot*	*reaction*	*A little*	*A lot*
3.	demoted at work	......	......	....	......	......
4.	not promoted when I hoped to be	......	......	....	......	......
5.	promoted	......	......	....	......	......
6.	laid off	......	......	....	......	......
7.	fired	......	......	....	......	......
8.	retired	......	......	....	......	......
9.	change in housework status	......	......	....	......	......

YOUR REACTION

other changes in work that had an impact on me:

10.

11.

CLOSE RELATIONSHIPS

1.	moved in with a mate or friend	......	......	....	......	......
2.	became engaged	......	......	....	......	......
3.	married	......	......	....	......	......
4.	separated	......	......	....	......	......
5.	divorced	......	......	....	......	......
6.	reunited with spouse or lover	......	......	....	......	......
7.	family member or significant person moved out	......	......	....	......	......
8.	family member or significant person moved in	......	......	....	......	......

Figure 3-10 /// 119

			YOUR REACTION		
	Negative		No	Positive	
	A little	A lot	reaction	A little	A lot
9. significant person or pet died	......	......	....	......	......
10. birth of a child	......	......	....	......	......
11. sexual difficulties	......	......	....	......	......
12. trouble with in-laws, family member, or housemate	......	......	....	......	......

other relationships
that had an impact on
me:

13.

14.

PHYSICAL/EMOTIONAL CHANGES

	Negative		No	Positive	
	A little	A lot	reaction	A little	A lot
1. became pregnant	......	......	....	......	......
2. abortion or miscarriage	......	......	....	......	......
3. started menstruating	......	......	....	......	......
4. menopause	......	......	....	......	......
5. serious illness or injury	......	......	....	......	......

CHANGE IN RESIDENCE

	Negative		No	Positive	
	A little	A lot	reaction	A little	A lot
1. moved to a new residence (home or institution)	......	......	....	......	......
2. remodeled a home	......	......	....	......	......
3. lost a home due to fire, flood, or disaster	......	......	....	......	......
4. took a vacation	......	......	....	......	......

(continued)

Figure 3–10 (continued)

	Negative		No	Positive	
	A little	A lot	reaction	A little	A lot

other residence changes that had an impact on me:

5.

6.

FINANCES

1. inherited or won a large amount of money ....

2. lost money or property ....

3. took out a loan or mortgage ....

4. have less money due to added financial responsibilities or cut in income ....

5. went on or off subsidy (welfare, scholarship, etc.) ....

6. got a big salary raise ....

7. started buying a large purchase on the installment plan ....

other financial situations that had an impact on me:

Figure 3-10 /// *121*

		YOUR REACTION			
	Negative		No	Positive	
	A little	A lot	reaction	A little	A lot
8.					
9.					

SUDDEN CHALLENGE

		Negative		No	Positive	
1.	unwanted pregnancy	......	......	....	......	......
2.	premature birth	......	......	....	......	......
3.	emergency hospitaliza- tion or surgery	......	......	....	......	......
4.	involuntary placement in an institution (rehabilitation hospi- tal, jail, nursing home)	......	......	....	......	......
5.	flood or other natural disaster	......	......	....	......	......
6.	holidays	......	......	....	......	......
7.	sudden move to new residence	......	......	....	......	......
8.	outstanding personal achievement	......	......	....	......	......
9.	suicide attempt	......	......	....	......	......
10.	accident	......	,,,,,,	....	......	......
11.	rape or other assault	......	......	....	......	......
12.	robbed	......	......	....	......	......
13.	suddenly overcame an illness	......	......	....	......	......

other sudden challenges
that had an impact on
me:

14.

15.

(continued)

Figure 3–10 (continued)

OTHER CHALLENGES

(List other challenges here that may be influencing your health. For example, *fears* of: losing money or losing a significant person, or decreasing or increasing your social activities):

1.

2.

3.

4.

5.

6.

7.

Now take a look back at the *Negative—A lot* column. If you have one or more events listed, you may wish to conduct an active grieving around that event. Also, take a look at the *No Reaction* column. See where you checked No Reaction and ask yourself for each check: "Is it reasonable for me to have no reaction to this event?" "If I allowed myself to have a reaction, what reaction would it be?" If you do come up with a reaction, you may also want to do some active grieving around that event. In that case, turn to the section on grieving in Chapter 4.

Figure 3-11 /// 123

**Figure 3-11   General Directions for Visualization
Self-Healing Technique**

Step 1:   Put yourself in a deeply relaxed, receptive state. Relax your body, close your eyes, and concentrate on picturing in your mind the healing process.

Step 2:   See the healing images clearly and in tiny detail. Concentrate on these images. Gently bring your mind back to these images. Change your images in any way that seems right to you at that time.

Step 3:   Become aware of what you are thinking and feeling as you picture these healing images. Allow any feeling that comes to you to be experienced. They are all part of the healing process. Try to get in touch with any negative feelings you have about healing and becoming well. Concentrate on these negative feelings or thoughts, and explore and challenge them. Give yourself permission to confront and successfully deal with your negative feelings and thoughts.

Step 4:   Stand by your right to heal yourself and be well. Tell yourself in words or think the thought, "I deserve to be well."

Step 5:   Trust and believe that you can heal yourself. Give this process an honest chance to work.

Figure 3–12   Visualization for People Who Have Cancer

Step 1:   Put yourself in a deeply relaxed state. Close your eyes, relax your body. You are deeply relaxed.

Step 2:   Picture your cancer: what do you see?

Step 3:   Allow yourself to experience whatever feelings occur to you as you visualize your cancer. Concentrate on making the image of the cancer vivid.

Step 4:   When you have the cancer vividly in mind, imagine an army of healthy white blood cells carrying off the malignant cells. The cancer cells are losing their power and are being overcome by your healthy white blood cells.

Step 5:   Picture the cancer cells being flushed out of your system by the healthy white blood cells. Your cancer is getting smaller and smaller and has less and less ability to harm you.

Step 6:   Picture any other treatments or methods you are using to fight your cancer coming in to help your white blood cells.

Step 7:   Your white blood cells are becoming more and more powerful, and they work together with your other treatments and methods. The cancer cells are getting ever weaker and more and more confused. The cancer cells are getting more and more easy to destroy.

Step 8:   Allow yourself to be well and to conquer your cancer. Allow yourself to experience the good feeling of mastering your body.

Step 9:   (Optional) Ask yourself, "Why did I need my cancer in the first place?" Gradually explore this question, and do not force the answer. It will come to you. Once you find the answer, trust yourself to find a healthier way of meeting that need.

Figure 3–13 /// 125

Figure 3–13   Visualization Exercise for Constant Worry and Fear

---

Step 1:   Put yourself in a deeply relaxed state. Close your eyes, and relax. You are deeply relaxed.

Step 2:   Think of the things you have been worrying about, and fear will happen. Slowly let these images pass before you. If at any point you become anxious or fearful, stop the image, and relax your body. Any time you want to stop the image, you can. You are in complete control of your images.

Step 3:   Continue to let the images pass before you. Say hello to each, let yourself realize these are images you have created, and so they are part of you. Experience any negative thoughts or feelings you have about giving up these worries and fears.

Step 4:   Picture how well you would be if you were to give up these worries and fears.

Step 5:   Bring back the images of fear and worry one by one. Picture yourself waving good-bye to each one. Allow yourself to experience whatever feeling you have as you wave good-bye.

Step 6:   Slowly let the images fade, realizing that you have said good-bye to your worry and fear. Allow yourself to feel at peace now as the worries and fears leave you.

Figure 3–14   Visualization Exercise for People With Glaucoma

---

Step 1:   Put yourself in a deeply relaxed state. Close your eyes and relax. You are deeply relaxed.

Step 2:   Think of things you do not want to see—things that trouble you. Let those images pass before your eyes. Allow yourself to experience whatever thoughts or feelings you have about those things that trouble you. If you find yourself tensing up, stop the images, and relax your body. You are in complete control of your images at all times.

Step 3:   When you feel relaxed and ready to proceed, distance yourself from the images of things that have troubled you. Believe that these things cannot touch you unless you allow them to. Experience peace and calm.

Step 4:   Picture yourself being good to your eyes. Picture yourself loving and caring for your eyes.

Step 5:   Picture large sponges soaking up excess fluid around your eyes, and the pressure is draining away. Now picture yourself gently helping the sponges to clear your eyes.

Step 6:   Believe that you can heal your eyes. Allow yourself to feel good about your ability to heal yourself.

Figure 3–15   Visualization Exercise for "Hot" (Infected or Irritated) Areas or Organs

---

Step 1:   Put yourself in a relaxed, receptive state. Close your eyes, relax, and be comfortable. Your body is deeply relaxed.

Step 2:   Visualize the area in your body that feels hot and uncomfortable. Vividly picture that area of your body.

Step 3:   Visualize the heat leaving that area. Replace the warmth in that area with cool, clear air. Every time you exhale, that part of your body is feeling cooler and cooler. Each time you exhale, you remove more and more heat. Watch the heat actually leave that area and be replaced by refreshing coolness.

Step 4:   Repeat this process until the "hot" area feels cool.

Figure 3-16 /// 127

Figure 3-16   Consulting Your Own Health Adviser

Step 1:   Choose a time when you are not rushed. Relax your body completely using a relaxation exercise, and find a quiet place to meditate.

Step 2:   Totally focus on visualizing your health adviser in your mind's eye. In your mind, go to a place where you are comfortable and at peace. Go to a high mountain, a warm beach, a peaceful lake. Look for your health adviser to appear to you. Wait peacefully, expectantly.

Step 3:   Let your imaginary health adviser come to you. Note what your adviser looks like. Get a strong feel for his or her size, shape, age, dress (if this applies).

Step 4:   Decide whether you want to touch your adviser or stand or sit a distance away.

Step 5:   Begin to talk to your adviser. Find out what kind of an adviser you have. Ask him or her questions about your health.

Step 6:   Realize that your conversation may seem silly or stilted at first, or it may seem perfectly natural. Whatever happens is O.K. Give yourself permission to carry on this conversation in whatever way it occurs.

Step 7:   When you have received answers to your questions, thank your adviser, and return to the here-and-now of present reality.

Step 8:   Allow yourself to feel good about your progress and what you have learned.

Step 9:   Begin to make plans for using the wisdom you have gained. Be confident that your internal adviser can be of help to you.

This exercise is not meant to be used when people are critically ill and require medical treatment. In that event, they should see a physician.

Figure 3–17   Directions for Using Positive Affirmations

Step 1:   Think of a positive statement about your ability to heal yourself. Some statements to consider are:

I, (your name), know that each time I think positively about healing, my body will be healing itself.

I, (your name), feel my body healing itself in a remarkable, wonderful way.

I, (your name), know my body can heal itself.

I, (your name), will work together with my body to heal and become well.

Step 2:   Write your chosen statement ten to twenty times a day. Be sure to say the statement aloud to yourself as you write it. Believe it.

Step 3:   If any doubts come to your mind while you are writing, assure yourself that you *can* heal yourself.

Figure 3-18 /// 129

Figure 3-18   Directions for the Cobra Posture

Reported Benefits: Tones ovaries, uterus, liver; provides relief for menstrual irregularities, constipation, and slipped discs.

Step 1:   Lie flat on your stomach on a rug or mat, with your legs together and your arms bent up toward your face.

Step 2:   Inhale *very* slowly while raising your chest and then your head slowly off the floor. Prop yourself up on your elbows. Tighten your buttocks muscles in your seat. Then relax and exhale slowly.

Step 3:   While inhaling slowly, and keeping your navel on the floor, raise the chest and head. Push with slow, steady pressure of your hands. Tighten the buttocks muscles of your seat, pulling your chest toward the ceiling and arching your back vertebra by vertebra. Let the top of your head reach toward the wall behind you. Arch until you feel the pressure and pull. (Never arch to pain.)

Step 4:   Hold this position and your breath. Feel your strength and your blood energize your spine, your liver, and (if applicable) your uterus and ovaries.

Step 5:   Exhale very slowly while lowering each vertebra toward the floor.

Step 6:   Repeat steps two to five one to ten times.

Step 7:   Lie flat on the floor, with your face to one side. Allow yourself to feel the benefits of this posture.

Figure 3-19   Directions for the Complete Breath

Reported Benefits: increases vitality, soothes nerves, strengthens intestinal and abdominal muscles, relieves asthma, emphysema, shortness of breath.
It is not recommended for people who have peptic ulcer, hernia or hyper-thyroid.

Step 1:   Lie flat on your back with your knees up, feet flat on the floor slightly apart.

Step 2:   Place your hands lightly on your abdomen (stomach area).

Step 3:   Breathe in through your nose and expand only your abdomen. Watch your fingertips part.

Step 4:   Exhale and contract your abdomen. Feel your fingertips meet.

Step 5:   Practice this abdominal breath ten times. Do not strain. Let your breath flow in and out with ease. Listen to your breath go in and out. Visualize yourself relaxing as you exhale.

Step 6:   Place your hands on your rib cage.

Step 7:   Inhale very slowly, watching your fingertips part.

Step 8:   Very slowly exhale, contracting your rib cage.

Step 9:   Practice this diaphragm breath ten times.

Step 10:   Place your fingertips on your collarbones.

Step 11:   Raise your shoulders and inhale in the upper part of your chest. Feel your fingertips part.

Step 12:   Exhale slowly and then practice the upper breath ten times.

Step 13:   Place your hands, palms up, alongside your body.

Step 14:   Put the three breaths together. Inhale slowly, expanding first the abdomen, then the diaphragm, then the upper chest. Hold.

Step 15:   Exhale, contracting first the abdomen, then the rib cage, then the upper chest.

Step 16:   Repeat the Complete Breath, until you establish a comfortable, relaxing rhythm. Concentrate on what is happening in your body as you breathe. Feel the old, bad air leave your body. Feel the clean, fresh air healing your body as you breathe in. Notice how relaxed and calm you are becoming.

Figure 3-20 /// 131

Figure 3-20   Shoulder Stand

Reported Benefits: provides healing sleep, improves breathing, menstrual disorders, sinus congestion, varicose veins, and rheumatism, strengthens lower
back.
Not recommended for people with high blood pressure or enlarged liver, spleen,
or thyroid.

Step 1:   Fold a towel in half and place on the floor so that when you lie
down it covers the back of your shoulders and your neck.

Step 2:   Lie flat on your back on the towel.

Step 3:   Slide your palms underneath your buttocks, and bend your arms
to prop up your hips so you are balanced on your shoulders and
upper arms. Your elbows are on the floor, your knees are bent
over your head. Breathe shallowly and easily. Feel your release
from the effects of gravity, your internal organs are relaxing and
using the extra space available to them.

Step 4:   Slowly straighten your legs upward, pushing with your hands.
Keep your legs together. Point your toes. Find a comfortable
height to balance at. Support your back with your hands.

Step 5:   Hold this pose for as long as you are comfortable. Breathe slowly
and easily. Allow your legs to be steady and relaxed. Notice how
your body feels in this position. Allow your blood to move throughout your body in a healing way.

Step 6:   Lower your hips very slowly, rounding your back and returning
to lie flat on the floor.

Figure 3-21   The Lion Posture

Reported Benefits: Helps relieve sore throat and congestion from a cold

Step 1:   Sit on your heels.

Step 2:   Place your palms on your knees.

Step 3:   Fan out your fingers, stretching them as much as possible. You should feel a real stretch between your fingers.

Step 4:   Tense your whole body.

Step 5:   Roll your eyes upward while sticking your tongue out and down as far as it will go. Contract your throat muscles.

Step 6:   Exhale while forcing the breath out and loudly saying *"Ahhhh!"*

Step 7:   Repeat one to seven times. Increase the tensing motion. Feel your blood taking away the swelling and soreness from your throat and bringing fresh, soothing blood to it.

Figure 3-22 /// 133

Figure 3-22   Directions for Practicing Laying on of Hands

Step 1:   Sit quietly, alone in a comfortable place.

Step 2:   Close your eyes and notice what is going on inside your body. How are you breathing? Where is there tension? Where is there comfort? What sensations do you feel? Center yourself, and become attuned to your environment.

Step 3:   Slowly open your eyes, and rub the palms of your hands together quickly for a few seconds.

Step 4:   Hold your hands several inches apart, palms facing. Allow your shoulders, arms, and hands to relax. Feel the energy passing between your hands. Experiment by holding your palms farther apart and closer together. Notice where you feel the most energy. Sense what shape the energy force has.

Step 5:   Lie on your back on the floor with your knees bent. Close your eyes, and relax your body. Again, rub your palms together quickly, then place them a few inches apart until you feel energy passing between them.

Step 6:   Place your arms around yourself. Hold yourself in a comfortable, healing way. After a few minutes, you may want to pretend you are being held, rather than holding. Stay in this position as long as you feel comfortable.

Step 7:   Place your hands at your sides. Keep your eyes closed, and note how you feel different and where you feel different. Allow yourself to make this experience part of you.

Step 8:   Slowly stretch, open your eyes, and sit up.

Figure 3-23   Directions for Practicing Laying on of Hands on Others

---

Step 1:   Decide together whether you will stand, sit, or assume different positions. The one who is laying on hands may decide to kneel beside the other who lies down. Experiment with the comfort of different positions. Neither of you can work effectively if uncomfortable. Change positions at any time during the session.

Step 2:   Tell the person you are working with to close his or her eyes and focus deep inside their body, to note where there is tension or comfort and to pay attention to breathing patterns.

Step 3:   Rub your hands together quickly, face the palms together a few inches apart, and feel the energy flow between them.

Step 4:   Hold your hands several inches from the person's body. Move from head to toes, noting places which feel stronger, weaker, tighter, looser, congested, clear, cool, warm, numb, tingling, and so on.

Step 5:   Choose one or more places you feel can benefit from your energy.

Step 6:   Quickly rub your hands together, feel the energy between them, and place your hands on the place or places you have chosen, keeping your hands several inches above the body. Relax your hands, and be open to energy transfer. Feel the energy flowing from your hands to the other person's body. Leave your hands where you have placed them for as long as you feel a connection. Watch the other person for more relaxation or deeper breathing. It is better to work for too short a time than for too long. You can repeat the session a few days later if necessary.

Step 7:   Once you have removed your hands, have the person lie still for five to ten minutes with eyes closed.

Step 8:   If the other person complains that the pain has moved to another body part, direct the energy through the body, and smooth it out past his or her feet, using a stroking motion.

Figure 3–24 /// *135*

Figure 3–24   Some Warming-up and Cooling-down Exercises

These exercises will prepare your body for conditioning. Stretch *very* slowly, do *not* bounce to attain or maintain a position. Let your body slowly stretch as far as is comfortable for you. Gradually increase the stretch. Hold each position for 15 to 30 seconds.

1. Squat on the floor, knees bent, feet flat on the floor. Hold on to a drawer or something that is at your arm level when they are relaxed in front of your legs. Hold the squat for 30 seconds if possible. Now stand up.

2. Bend over at the waist, bending your knees slightly. Let gravity take your arms slowly closer and closer to the floor. Relax, and let the upper part of your body stretch. Hold each position for up to 30 seconds.

3. Stand an arm's length from a wall with your right side facing the wall. Place your right hand on the wall for support. Slowly grasp your left ankle with your left hand and very slowly pull your foot up and back until the heel touches your buttocks. Be sure to lean forward from the waist as you lift. Feel the stretch in the upper front part of your leg. Repeat, with your left side facing the wall, grasping the right ankle. Allow the muscles of your upper front legs to stretch for 15 to 30 seconds.

4. Sit on the floor with one of your legs extended in front of you, the other leg bent with the heel close to your buttocks. Slowly slide your hands down the extended leg until you are in a steady stretch for 15 to 30 seconds, then let go of your leg and slowly slide your elbows on the floor. Rest in this position for 15 to 30 seconds; pay attention to the blood flow in your body and the stretching of your muscles. Repeat the exercise with your other leg extended in front of you.

5. Sit on the floor and place the soles of your feet together. Place your hands around your feet. Very slowly, move your head in a controlled stretch toward your feet. Hold the stretch for up to 30 seconds, relaxing your back and groin muscles into the stretch.

6. Sit on the floor, with your legs spread as wide apart as you can. Slowly lean forward from the waist, reaching toward an imaginary spot on the floor directly in front of you. Relax your back and groin muscles in the stretch for 15 to 30 seconds. Now slowly move your arms and upper body toward your left leg. Stretch your chin toward your left leg in an even, controlled stretch; hold for 15 to 30 seconds. Now slowly move your arms and upper body toward your right leg. Stretch your chin toward your right leg in an even, controlled stretch; hold for 15 to 30 seconds.

(continued)

Figure 3-24 (continued)

---

7.   Prop your left leg up on the back or arm of a sofa or outside on a railing or fence. Be sure the prop gives you adequate support. Bend your nose toward your left knee in a slow, controlled stretch. Let the muscles of your left leg, arms, and back relax into the stretch. Hold this position for 15 to 30 seconds.

8.   Stand facing a wall, about three feet away from it. Place both hands on the wall. Slowly lean forward toward the wall, keeping your back straight and your heels flat on the floor. Bend your elbows to your hands. Hold the position for 15 to 30 seconds, then slowly push with the palm of your hands and straighten your arms. Feel the effects of the stretch in your lower legs and calves and in your arms and chest.

9.   Stand with your arms extended forward and your palms touching. Slowly bring your arms back to shoulder level, as if pushing against an invisible force. Open your chest, and breathe in and out deeply. Clasp your hands behind your back, arms extended. Inhale deeply, and pull your shoulders back, your upper chest toward the ceiling. Tighten your buttocks muscles and reach for the wall behind you gradually with your head. Then bend forward, raising your arms (still clasped and extended) over your head. Stretch your arms on additional 1/2 inch. Exhale, and return to upright standing position. Keep hands clasped together, but bend elbows loosely. Slowly rotate, twisting your hips, spine, and head to the left, then rotate slowly to the right. Drop your arms, and relax, feeling the increased circulation to your lungs and spine.

10. Kneel on your hands and knees in a stable position. Slowly make your back concave, and bring your chin down to your hands. Push with your palms, straightening your arms. Now round your back as much as possible. These two movements should look like a cat when it stretches. Very slowly bring your left knee to meet your forehead; hold for several seconds, then extend your right knee behind you, pointing your toe. Stretch with your extended leg and toe. Hold for 10 seconds. Repeat with right leg. Relax by sitting back on your heels and placing your arms on your thighs. Allow your body to feel the benefits from stretching.

11. Lie on your back. Raise your knees and clasp your hands under your knees. Gently rock back and forth on your rounded spine. Do not roll back too far on your neck. Feel your back round and feel the massaging action on the spine.

Figure 3–25 /// 137

Figure 3–25   Sample Exercise Program for a 45-Year-Old Woman

---

First Segment: *Work up to* walking one mile in 15 minutes.

Second Segment: *Work up to* walking two miles in 30 minutes.

Third Segment: *Work up to* walking three miles in 45 minutes.

Fourth Segment: (remain in this segment for *at least* eight to ten weeks) Complete stretching exercises (Figure 3–24). Jog slowly, stopping to walk when you are breathing too fast to jog and talk to someone at the same time; do this for 20 minutes three times a week. Walk last tenth of a mile. Complete stretching and cooling-down exercises.

Fifth Segment: Complete stretching exercises before and after jogging. Jog for 20 minutes four or five times a week. Walk last tenth of a mile.

Sixth Segment: Complete stretching exercises before and after jogging. Jog for 30 minutes three to five times a week. Walk last tenth of a mile.

Seventh Segment: Complete stretching exercises before and after jogging. Increase jogging time if comfortable doing so, or remain at 30 minutes three to five times a week. Remember to walk last tenth of a mile.

Figure 3–26   Exercises for an Older Person

---

1. Stand comfortably erect, with your feet about a foot apart. Place your hands on your hips. Inhale deeply, and rotate your hips in a wide circular motion. Exhale. Continue to inhale, rotate your hips, and exhale seven times. Allow your pelvis to do all the motion. Try not to lead with your shoulders or head. Relax for a few minutes after completing the seven rotations, then do seven rotations in the opposite direction. If you need support, hold on to a chair. When you have finished, feel how your circulation has improved to your pelvis, spine, lower back, and legs.

2. Lie flat on your back. Inhale and slowly bend your right knee toward your chest. Clasp both hands around your knee, and hold it as close to your chest as is comfortable. Inhale deeply, holding your knee, while slowly counting to seven. As you exhale, slowly allow your leg to straighten and return to the floor. Experience the new flow of blood to your lower back, buttocks, and legs. Allow yourself to feel the release of tension and tightness in your abdomen, groin, and pelvis.

3. Stand comfortably erect, with your feet about a foot apart, or lie flat on the floor. Inhale slowly as you stretch your arms high overhead. Feel the stretch as you unlock your chest. Extend your right fingertips as far as possible while pushing down with your heels. Allow yourself to feel a controlled stretch down the right-hand side of your body. Repeat while extending your left fingertips and pushing down with your heels. Repeat, extending each side seven times. Lie comfortably at rest, breathing deeply. Feel the benefits to your breathing and circulation.

4. Sit in a firm, comfortable chair. Relax, and let your head drop onto your chest. Breathe comfortably, and gently rotate your head to your left shoulder, then around to the right shoulder. Rotate your head in a complete circle seven times, then rotate in the opposite direction seven times. Allow all the tension and stiffness to go out of your head.

5. Lie on your back, with your knees bent and the soles of your feet close to your buttocks. While breathing in a deep, relaxed way, press your tailbone firmly to the floor, then slowly rock your pelvis back, pressing the small of your back to the floor. Repeat this movement seven times. Relax, and feel the increased relaxation in your lower back, pelvis, and legs.

Figure 3-26 /// 139

6. Lie on your back, and extend your arms straight out at your shoulders. Bend your knees and draw them up toward your left arm while turning your head slowly toward your right arm. Then slowly roll your lower body toward your right arm while turning your head slowly toward your left arm. Exhale when it feels comfortable to do so. Repeat this motion several times on each side, then lie flat, and feel the effect of this exercise on your muscles and joints, your neck, hips, spine, chest, and abdomen.

7. Sit with your legs together, extended in front of you. Inhale deeply and slowly raise your arms above your head, stretching your fingers toward the ceiling. As you exhale, slowly reach your hands down the front of your legs toward your toes. Let your head, neck, and back relax. Breathe easily and hold yourself in a controlled stretch for a slow count of ten. Slowly raise your head, and sit up comfortably. Repeat several more times, then relax, and feel the benefits in your arms, neck, lower back, and the back of your legs.

8. Complete the exercise described in Figure 3-18.

9. Complete the second exercise in Figure 3-23.

NOTES

1. Donald M. Vickery. *Life Plan for Your Health*. Reading, Mass.: Addison-Wesley, 1978, pp. 10-11.
2. Walter W. Rosser. "Screening in family medicine: the current situation," *Journal of Family Practice* 6, no. 3 (1978), pp. 503-510.
3. Paul S. Frame and Stephen J. Carlson. "A critical review of periodic health screening using specific screening criteria," *Journal of Family Practice* 2, no. 1-4 (1975).
4. John J. Calabro and Bertram A. Malta. "Ankylosing spondylitis," *New England Journal of Medicine* 282, no. 11 (1970), pp. 606-610.
5. David S. Guzick. "Efficacy of screening for cervical cancer: a review," *American Journal of Public Health* 68, no. 2 (1978), pp. 125-134.
6. Jon J. Dutton. "Procedures in family practice: sigmoidoscopy as a periodic screening test," *Journal of Family Practice* 7, no. 5 (1978), pp. 1041-1046.
7. Wilfred H. Palmer and Christine L. White. "The electrocardiogram in ambulatory medical practice," *Journal of Family Practice* 8, no. 1, pp. 29-35.
8. Donald L. Wiener et al. "Exercise stress testing: correlation among history of angina, S-T segment response and prevalence of coronary artery disease in the coronary artery surgery study (CASS)," *New England Journal of Medicine* 3-1, no. 5 (1979), pp. 230-235.
9. Richard H. Gold. "Indications and risk-benefit of mammography," *Journal of Family Practice* 8, no. 6 (1979), pp. 1135-1140.
10. Abraham B. Bergman. "The menace of mass screening," *American Journal of Public Health* 67, no. 7 (1977), pp. 601-602.
11. Rudolf J. Napodano. "The functional heart murmur: a wastebasket diagnosis," *Journal of Family Practice* 4, no. 4 (1977), pp. 637-639.
12. Herbert L. Abrahms. "The 'overutilization' of x-rays," *New England Journal of Medicine* 300, no. 21 (1979), pp. 1213-1216.
13. "University group diabetes program: a study of the effects of hypoglycemic agents on vascular complications in patients with adult onset diabetes," *Journal of the American Medical Association*, supplement 2, no. 1 (1970).
14. David L. Sackett. "Screening for early detection of disease: to what purpose?" *Bulletin of the New York Academy of Medicine* 51, no. 1, pp. 39-52.
15. Donald A. F. Nelson, et al. "Emergency room misuse by medical assistance patients in a family practice residency," *Journal of Family Practice* 8, no. 2 (1979), pp. 341-345.
16. Vickery, *Life Plan*, pp. 195-263.
17. Robert S. Galen. "False-positives," *Lancet* (Nov. 2, 1974), p. 1081.
18. Sackett, "Screening."
19. Robert Rodale. "Learn your signs of health," *Prevention* (November 1978), p. 22.
20. "How's your blood pressure doing?" *Prevention* (January, 1975), pp. 81-90.

21. Mike Samuels and Hal Bennett. *The Well Body Book*. New York: Random House, 1973, pp. 180-181.
22. Vickery, *Life Plan*, p. 6.
23. Marie M. Seedor. *The Physical Assessment*. New York: Teachers College Press, 1974, pp. 79, 89-99.
24. Vickery, *Life Plan*, pp. 165-172.
25. H. V. Wyatt. "Polio immunization: benefits and risks," *Journal of Family Practice* 7, no. 3 (1978), pp. 469-474.
26. Joy Gardner. "Vaccines: friend or foe," *Well-Being*, no. 42, pp. 26-34.
27. Thomas H. Holmes and R. H. Rahe. "The social readjustment rating scale," *Journal of Psychosomatic Research* 2 (1967), pp. 213-218.
28. Samuels and Bennett. *The Well Body Book*, pp. 1-2.
29. Adelaide Bry. *Directing the Movies of Your Mind*. New York: Harper & Row, 1978, pp. 64-102.
30. Harvey Mindess. "The sense in humor," *Saturday Review* (April 21, 1971), pp. 10-12.
31. R. John Wakeman and Jerold Z. Kaplan. "An experimental study of hypnosis in painful burns," *The American Journal of Clinical Hypnosis* 21, no. 1 (1978), pp. 3-9.
32. Paul Sacerdote. "Teaching self-hypnosis to patients with chronic pain," *Journal of Human Stress* 4, no. 2 (1978), pp. 18-21.
33. Dabney M. Ewin. "Relieving suffering—and pain—with hypnosis," *Geriatrics* 33, no. 6 (1978), pp. 87-89.
34. "Self hypnosis and healing," *Prevention* (September, 1977), pp. 64-70.
35. Zahourek, Rothlyn. "Use of relaxation and hypnotic techniques in the care of the disturbed patient." A one-day workshop for nurses given by the College of Nursing, Downstate Medical Center, SUNY, Brooklyn, New York, November 1, 1978.
36. Areed F. Barabasy and Christopher M. McGeorge. "Biofeedback, mediated biofeedback and hypnosis in peripheral vasodilation training," *The American Journal of Clinical Hypnosis* 21, no. 1 (July 1978), pp. 28-33.
37. Lawrence LeShan. "You can fight for your life," *Emotional Factors in the Causation of Cancer*. New York: M. Evans and Co., 1977, pp. 88-89.
38. Bry, *Movies of Your Mind*, pp. 91-93.
39. Ibid., pp. 98-99.
40. Ibid., pp. 94-95.
41. Irving Oyle. *Time, Space and Mind*. Millbrae, Calif.: Celestial Arts, 1976.
42. Sonya Herman. *The Assertive Nurse* 1, no. 3, p. 5.
43. Theodosia Gardner. "Yoga therapy." In *The Practical Encyclopedia of Natural Healing*, pp. 537-552.
44. Ibid.
45. Jess Stearn. *Yoga, Youth, and Reincarnation*. New York: Bantam, 1965, p. 317.
46. John Diamond. *BK Behavioral Kinesiology*. New York: Harper & Row, 1979, p. 2.
47. Ibid., p. 25.

48. Ibid., p. 17.
49. Ibid., pp. 21–22.
50. Chellis Glendinning. "Laying on of hands." In *The Holistic Health Handbook*, Berkeley, Calif.: And/Or Press, 1978, pp. 180–182.
51. Dolores Krieger. *American Journal of Nursing* 79, no. 4 (1979), pp. 660–662.
52. Dolores Krieger. *The Therapeutic Touch*. Englewood Cliffs, N.J.: Prentice Hall, 1979.
53. Janet Macral. "Therapeutic touch in practice," *American Journal of Nursing* 79, no. 4 (1979), pp. 664–665.
54. Donald B. Ardell. *High Level Wellness*. Emmaus, Pa.: Rodale, 1977, pp. 145–146.
55. Ibid., pp. 147 and 159.
56. Samuels and Bennett. *The Well Body Book*, pp. 98–99.
57. The President's Council on Physical Fitness and Sports. *An Introduction to Running, One Step At a Time*. Washington, D.C.: HEW. n.d.
58. "How different sports rate in promoting physical fitness," *Resident and Staff Physician* (August 1976), p. 44.
59. Diamond, *BK Behavioral Kinesiology*, pp. 40–42.
60. "How different sports rate," pp. 44–49.
61. Diamond, *BK Behavioral Kinesiology*, p. 42.
62. Mark Bricklin. "What readers want to know about fitness, figure and physique," *Prevention* (June, 1978), pp. 32–40.
63. Bronnie Krupis. *Running a Complete Guide*. New York: Dell, 1978, pp. 4–5.
64. Robert Rodale. "The pulse of your life," *Prevention* (March 1977), pp. 25–30.
65. Vickery, *Life Plan*, pp. 111–112.
66. Ardell, *High Level Wellness*, p. 90.
67. Vickery, *Life Plan*, pp. 109–111.
68. Ibid., p. 110.
69. Ibid., p. 111.
70. Ken Dychtwald, "Exercises for lifelong health and well-being," *Prevention* (January 1979), pp. 79–88.
71. Thomas DeCarlo, Lawrence Castiglione, and Melmet Cavusoglu. "A program of balanced physical fitness in the preventive care of elderly ambulatory patients," *Journal of the American Geriatric Society* 25 (1977), pp. 331–334.

4

Feeling Good

This chapter focuses on ways you can help yourself to feel good, through the use of stress reduction methods such as relaxation exercises, yoga, self-hypnosis, creative visualization, centering, meditation, massage, baths, humor, dance, music, poetry, and inner shouting. Feeling good also deals with ways of reducing pain, getting rid of unwanted symptoms, and facing situations where stress cannot be reduced because one has to deal with them. This entails being able to take assertive positions such as learning how to control anxiety, fear, and anger while standing up for one's rights; disagreeing; expressing anger; dealing with the anger of others; handling a putdown; asking for a legitimate workload, legitimate salary, or legitimate health care. It also means spreading out life changes and learning to anticipate stressful events. Feeling good about oneself and life situations also comes from learning to grieve for changes, losses, and separations; unresolved losses lead to illness processes such as depression and to loss of optimism about the future. A final aspect to be discussed in this chapter is sleep; without adequate rest and sleep, no one can feel good or function well.

STRESS AND STRESS REDUCTION

Selye defines stress as "the nonspecific response of the body to any demand made upon it" [1]. Our bodies are built to withstand stress and to use adaptive functions to reestablish a comfortable state. If we are exposed to too much stress over a long period of time, we can develop tension, insecurity, frustration, headaches, ulcers, heart attacks, high blood pressure, depression (or other forms of what is called mental illness), suicidal thoughts or actions, bowel irritations, diabetes, and assorted skin disorders [2, 3]. Friedman and Rosenman claim there is one "type" of individual (Type A), who has a specific personality and behavior pattern that *brings on* stress by being excessively competitive, aggressive, impatient, and by having "a harrying sense of time urgency" [4].

Figure 4-1 indicates signs of nonhelpful stress, including some Type A behaviors. Some people seem to thrive on stress; they can adapt to difficult situations and know when to quit if there is no remedy to a problem. It is *not* the seeming stressfulness of a situation that is the problem; it is the *person's reaction* to situations that creates difficulties. A study of 800 executives showed that there was no correlation between a change in anxiety level and salary, number of hours worked, or number of hours spent commuting. What *was* experienced as stressful by these executives was *their* lack of satisfaction with their job, their *perception* of job stress, and their reported health problems [5].

Finances and family squabbles can be more stressful than work for some people. Others who are overeducated for their jobs or who have no challenge in their lives can still be under a great deal of stress [6]. You need to identify what is stressful for *you*. Figure 4-2 can be used for this purpose. In addition, refer back to Figure 3-10 to see what changes may be creating stress for you at this time; use this in conjunction with Figure 4-3 to find ways of reducing stressful life changes.

There are many questions yet to be answered about stress and its effect on wellness. For example, is it possible that stress can be categorized into positive and negative types? Can it be that stress *perceived* as a challenge or as change toward a more creative, fulfilling life is positive or wellness-enhancing, whereas change that stunts growth or that results in the individual feeling exploited or hampered is perceived as negative and opposed to wellness? If this model works, how can we learn to assess positive and negative sources better? How can we learn to intervene so stress does not lead to illness?

Relaxation Exercises

Once sources of stress have been identified, steps can be taken to reduce their effects. One way is through regular practice of relaxation exercises. There are many different kinds of relaxation exercises: the total body relaxation, and specific kinds of exercises for tension in various body parts. In general, all need to be practiced regularly, preferably every day, if full benefits are to be derived. Those who are unfamiliar with relaxing body parts will need regular practice. It is not sufficient to wait until high tension is noted in the body and then practice the exercise; exercises should be mastered prior to the time they are really needed. Once you are able to relax muscles during low-stress times, you can transfer that learning to high-stress situations. For example, if you practice the Total Body Relaxation Exercise (see Figure 4-4) you can use it on the way to, and even during, situations you perceive as high-stress ones. The Total Body Relaxation Exercise can also be used to relax prior to going to sleep. The Contracting and Relaxing Exercise (Figure 4-5 [7]) can be used if you have difficulty knowing the difference between contracted and relaxed muscles. You can rate yourself from 1 to 100 in terms of tenseness. As you practice the exercise, you can rerate yourself. With practice, you will be more and more able to rate your tenseness correctly.

There are other relaxation exercises for specific body parts. Figure 4-6 gives directions for relaxing tense facial muscles; Figure 4-7 for relaxing stiff back and shoulders; Figure 4-8 for shoulder-neck tension [8]; Figure 4-9 for relaxing the body through foot relaxation [9]; and Figure 4-10 for general unwinding through alternate-nostril breathing [10, 11]. Figure 4-11 gives exercises for those who need to reduce tension while at home or at work.

Yoga

Many of the relaxation exercises given above are based on yoga. Most of the yoga exercises presented in Chapter 3, Being Fit, will also produce release of tension and relaxation; stretching exercises are especially useful for this. Those not presented in Chapter 3 or 4 can be found in basic yoga texts; these include The Chest Expander, Cat Stretch, The Pendulum, The Hugging Exercise, Invisible Wings.

Self-Hypnosis

What is Hypnosis?

Hypnosis is not a deep sleep. It is a wakeful state of deep relaxation, with an alteration in the conscious level of thinking and remembering, and an increase in the ability to focus in on a particular situation. Whenever a person concentrates better and is in a relaxed state, you can say hypnosis is occurring. *Hypnosis is a heightened state of awareness.*

Why do you talk about "self-hypnosis"?

All hypnosis is self-hypnosis. In some cases, the person uses a hypnotist as a guide, but the person's responses always remain under his or her control. If anything, people gain *more* control over what happens to them while undergoing hypnosis, and they are very alert and focused on what they are trying to change [12].

If people are more in control when hypnotized, why do stage hypnotists get people to do such silly things?

People who are ready to agree to do what the stage hypnotist asks go onto the stage, and they agree to be subjects and to be performers. The others in the audience do not agree to be performers. The stage hypnotist sets the conditions and suggests how the audience participant will act, just as people who use hypnotism set the conditions and suggest how they will act. In the latter case, people will decline any invitation to act like a rooster when they are there to learn how to quit smoking, stop bleeding, feel less pain, or whatever.

Can a hypnotist make me do something I don't want to do?

No. No one will do anything under hypnosis that is against his or her principles or carry out a suggestion unless it is acceptable [13].

I overeat when I'm tense and nervous. If I use hypnosis, won't I develop other problems when I stop overeating?

No. This is a carryover from the old mechanical idea of how people operated. Today, we use an open systems model to understand behavior and find that deep-seated difficulties are not aggravated when superficial problems are cleared up. If anything, the sense of mastery you get from controlling your eating habits may carry over to other aspects of your life.

Is there any danger in practicing self-hypnosis?

No, either you will master the skill and produce results or you will have no results. When there is physical pain, it is wise to consult a health practitioner first to make sure what the underlying causes of the pain are. With self-hypnosis you can reduce pain to a feeling of pressure. Thus, if the pressure continues after hypnosis, this is a sign that the underlying problem is still there [14].

If hypnosis is so useful, why don't doctors use it more often?

Many doctors don't use it because they have not been educated to do so, and they hold many of the misconceptions held by the general public. It also takes time to use hypnosis effectively [15]. There are, however, several periodicals and two national professional societies for health practitioners who use hypnosis; addresses for the societies are:

> The Society for Clinical and Experimental Hypnosis
> 353 W. 57th St.
> New York, New York

> The American Society for Clinical Hypnosis
> 800 Washington Avenue, S.E.
> Minneapolis, Minnesota

Hypnosis really is an unusual state, isn't it?

Not at all. You have probably hypnotized yourself thousands of times. Daydreaming is a state of hypnosis. You have also hypnotized yourself when you concentrated intently on a book, movie, television program, work project, or when experiencing strong emotion. During these times you slipped into a trance state.

Why is it important whether you use positive or negative suggestion?

Suggestion is used all the time in health care situations but usually of the negative kind. For example, health care practitioners are often quite unaware that the subconscious mind hears at all times, even during sleep or unconsciousness due to injury, illness, or anesthesia.

Adverse suggestions, such as "She'll never recover from this," or "It's malignant, the patient doesn't have a chance," or "You can't be helped, you will have to learn to live with the condition" (this last comment seems innocuous, but taken literally it means the client will die if she loses the symptom) are not only heard, but are frequently acted on by clients [16].

Positive suggestions have more force and effectiveness than do negative ones. It is wise to eliminate negative words such as not, don't, won't, or can't. "I will not feel tension tomorrow" is a negative suggestion, whereas, "I will feel comfortable and confident during the interview tomorrow" is a positive one. Permissive suggestions ("You can") often work better when they are repeated. Although repetition of positive suggestions is important, time must be allowed for the idea to take effect ("My comfort is gradually increasing" instead of "I am totally comfortable"). Suggestions are usually more effective when only one or two ideas are used; bombarding oneself with numerous suggestions only dilutes the force of all of them. Since hypnosis is a relaxed state with heightened focus, be sure only one or two ideas are suggested for focus.

Are there any people who should not attempt self-hypnosis?

Perhaps 80 to 90 percent of people can be hypnotized, but people who are severely emotionally disturbed, depressed, or suicidal probably need psychotherapy, not hypnosis. People who have psychosomatic illnesses yet deny any emotional component to their problem will not do well with hypnosis [17], nor will people who are neurologically impaired or mentally retarded [18].

Who is most hypnotizable?

People who are highly motivated to learn the technique, who are generally optimistic, willing to try something new, able to concentrate easily, receptive to rather than afraid of hypnosis, and have a good imagination are more likely to be hypnotized. Even people who do not have all these qualities can learn self-hypnosis if they are willing to practice the technique more frequently. There is a simple test that can be done to test the hypnotizability of a person. It is called the Eye-Roll Test, and it was developed by Dr. Herbert Spiegel, Clinical Professor of Psychiatry at Columbia University. Ninety-nine percent of hypnotizable subjects are able to perform this test [19]. Here is how the test works: Hold your head steady and look straight ahead. Keep your head in this spot, but look up toward the top of your head. (If you can see the ceiling you are looking toward the top of your head.) With your eyes still looking up, *slowly* close your eyelids. Then open your eyelids and let your eyes return to normal focus. If you can see the ceiling, self-hypnosis is possible.

Practicing Self-Hypnosis

Figure 4-12 gives basic instructions for self-hypnosis. It can be adapted for use when going to sleep. In this case, do not set a time limit to wake up (step 7). Instead, after step 11, give yourself the following suggestion: "I am relaxing more and more and becoming sleepier and sleepier. Within a few minutes, I will fall sound asleep and wake up refreshed in the morning." At this point, think no more about sleep. Rather, think of a pleasant experience [20].

Self-hypnosis can also be used to reduce stress related to smoking, drinking, overeating, taking harmful drugs, destructive anger, timidity, anxiety, allergies, itching, asthma, anger, study problems, and pain. The basic self-hypnotic state is induced (see Figure 4-12), but the person gives him- or herself different suggestions:

For my body, not for me but for my body, smoking (this harmful drug, destructive anger, anxiety, timidity, head symptom, drinking, overeating) is a poison. I need my body to live. To that degree I want to live, I will protect my body as I would protect (name of loved one) [21].

Suggestions for itching, allergies, and asthma would follow the same format with slight variation [22].
For itching:

Not for me, but for my body, this itch is damaging; it means my body is out of balance. To live comfortably, I need my body in balance. To the point I wish to live in comfort, I will itch when I choose to and at the body location I choose.

For allergies, asthma, or colds use the basic suggestion, but add:

If I choose to live this day symptom-free, I can, because I have power over my body. I can tell my nose when to get stuffed up and when not to. I can declare myself master of my body.

These suggestions are often more effective when used in conjunction with visualization; discussion of how to combine the two methods follows in the next section.

In order to benefit fully, you must practice the self-hypnosis technique (with the appropriate suggestion) once or twice every day until you have mastered it. At that point, you will be able to go into a deeply relaxed trance state by saying the cue words, such as "relax now."

Self-hypnosis is also useful in helping to slow the heart or breathing rate. In this instance, you take your pulse or respiration rate and then use the suggestion, "My pulse is slowing down a few beats a minute, and I'm relaxing" or "I am beginning to breathe more slowly and comfortably." After several moments, retake your pulse or respiration. If it has slowed sufficiently, think to yourself: "This is the heart rate (or pulse) I am comfortable with and want to remain at." This measure can be combined with creative visualization. For example, the heart can be visualized with blood slowing down as it enters and leaves the heart and as it passes through the arteries and veins of the body. Or, if breathing is to be slowed, picture your lungs slowly expanding and filling with clean air. As you breathe, picture your lungs expanding more slowly while filling up with clean, refreshing air.

Creative Visualization

The details of creative visualization were presented in Chapter 3. Creative visualization can also be used in conjunction with relaxation exercises and/or self-hypnosis. In either case, use your visual imagination to relax your body. People who have difficulty relaxing body parts may find creative visualization techniques of more use to them than muscle relaxation in reducing tension. Many people who use self-hypnotic techniques combine them with creative visualization.

One way of using visualization when all body muscles have been relaxed is to use your imagination to take yourself to a pleasant, relaxing place. Figure 4-13 gives the directions for a trip I used with a client who was in a wheelchair. You can develop your own "trips." First, it is important to get a clear idea regarding what settings you find relaxing and what is relaxing for you.

Creative visualization can also be combined with other relaxation methods for specific problems. If you feel tired at the end of the day, creative visualization can be used to overcome fatigue. The suggestion to use is: "You will begin to feel refreshed and full of energy." After using this suggestion, picture yourself playing a sport while full of vigor, or walking around full of energy. Carry this picture out to the fullest extent and hold it for three to four minutes. With this image, as with all visualizations for specific problems, the mental image represents the *desired* result. Thus, for obese people, the image would be of a very slim self [23].

A visualization to use to quit smoking:

Picture yourself in situations where you usually smoke. First see yourself with other people. You are surrounded by others. Picture the room completely clear of smoke. The air is clear and pleasant and you are enjoying the fresh air without coughing. You feel very relaxed and happy as you sit there enjoying your comfort and the fresh air. Now picture yourself alone, watching television or eating a meal. You see yourself as quite content to sit there with your hands free and nothing in your mouth. You see yourself enjoying the clear, fresh air and relaxing even more.

A visualization for the person who drinks:

Imagine yourself in a restaurant or at a cocktail party. You see yourself relaxed and enjoying the company even though you have had nothing to drink. You are at ease and order Perrier water with lime. Your friends look at you strangely and you hear yourself saying, "I feel like Perrier tonight." You picture yourself circulating and talking to other people. You are enjoying yourself and you feel at ease and relaxed. You notice other people are getting loud and beginning to slur their speech. You feel good that you are confident, relaxed, and enjoying yourself. Next, picture yourself alone and not drinking, yet feeling comfortable, relaxed, and confident [24].

For each specific problem, a relevant visualization can be devised using the format presented here.

Self-hypnosis can be combined with creative visualization to decrease study problems and enhance learning [25]. Students are taught to visualize themselves being successful at studying. (This image is first developed during deep relaxation.) Once students can conjure up this image easily, they "flash" this image before themselves at specified times during the day: upon awakening, right before going to sleep, prior to each meal, and whenever they feel bored, inactive, or negative. Students learn to "let their mind go blank" and then show a picture or movie of themselves being successful at studying or learning. Those who have difficulty visualizing a picture can be asked to "feel as if you are more successful." Suggestions students can learn to give themselves are: "I am studying more efficiently now." "I'm finding it more and more easy to learn." "I am finding a new ability to learn, recall information, and integrate this material with what I already know." "I am more able to treat failures as part of my road to success." "As my belief in my own ability increases, I see my potential for learning unlimited." In addition, students learn to say to themselves firmly three times before entering a study situation: "Concentrate and recall."

Centering

If illness is considered as energy imbalance, *centering* can help to reduce stress and bring the mind/body back into balance. Dr. John Diamond has studied the relationship between stress and cerebral balance. He suggests that people put their tongues against the roof of their mouth, "the tip about a quarter of an inch behind the upper front teeth" [26]. He refers to this spot as the "centering button." This spot seems to stimulate the thymus gland and weaken the effect of stress. (His theory can be tested by doing the muscle strength test, Chapter 2, pp. 32–33, shouting loudly at the person to introduce stress, redoing the muscle test, asking the client to push their centering button, and retesting.) Dr. Diamond has completed many clinical trials of the stress created by an imbalance and has found "that when the tongue is on the centering button, the cerebral hemispheres are balanced" [27]. Now this finding is of particular importance because many people are dominated by the left hemisphere of their cerebrum (brain) "which means they are trying to cope under too much stress" [28]. Left-sided dominance can lead to people who are caught in a verbal, intellectual struggle with themselves or their environment. Intuitive, aesthetic, and creative functions may be lost to them. By pushing their centering button, people can be helped to integrate both hemispheres in a coordinated, whole way. There are some other activities that tend to balance the two hemispheres of the brain: reading a poem in a rhythmic fashion, looking at pictures of pleasant landscapes, taking a vigorous walk while swinging one's arms, smiling while involving the muscles of the lower eyelid in the smile, looking at pictures of people who are smiling or who have their arms reaching out in a caring gesture, listening to a person who has a soothing voice, being near a waterfall or babbling brook, taking a shower, listening to classical music, listening to other natural sounds such as birds chirping or cats purring. (Tape recordings of these sounds will also work.) Maintaining good posture, and sitting in a hard-backed chair or on a firm seat or board, wearing low-heeled shoes that provide for good posture, swimming [29], and yogic and dance postures that enhance good posture will also be beneficial. Diamond also suggests that the Alexander posture be done daily. In this posture, you lie on your back with your knees bent and feet flat on the floor. It is important to have the body in alignment and to put some books under the head so the spine and neck are aligned [30]. Walking while pretending that there is an invisible cord that is fastened to the top of the head and through the spine to the floor that is pulling the chest out of the abdominal cavity and tilting the pelvis slightly forward will also improve posture and reduce stress on internal organs.

On the other hand, a phenomenon called "switching" occurs when certain activities are engaged in. In switching, the two hemispheres are not in balance, and there is a particular type of body confusion.

> People who are under constant stress may function with this switching pattern as their "normal" mode of behavior. The reciting of poetry in a rhythmic fashion, the viewing of landscape paintings, enhanced by thumping the thymus, should correct most imbalances. . . . [31].

There are daily activities that seem to lead to switching; try to avoid these situations and/or engage in the suggested centering activities. Some situations Diamond has found to precipitate switching are: weight lifting; bicycling; backhand strokes in tennis; wearing belts with buckles; partial dentures that have wires that cross the midline; metal-framed glasses; emotional states of hate, envy, suspicion, and fear; listening to someone who shows stress through their voice pattern; reading or hearing about murder, hijackings, floods, fires, or other disasters; rock music, or any music that does not flow on but stops at the end of a bar or measure; poor posture; sitting in a metal chair or a soft, comfortable chair when posture is poor; crossing legs or arms; wearing shoes that have too high heels or that make it difficult to maintain good posture [32].

Meditation

Meditation is a way of calming the mind and the body, letting in healing energy, and getting in touch with inner processes. There are many different meditation techniques. Figure 4-14 gives directions for one approach that is particularly suited to enhancing healing and self-respect.

A characteristic of meditative postures is that the spine is kept straight. Bodily posture has been shown both to reflect and to influence the inner state of the mind. By being absolutely still, even inexperienced meditators can lower their blood pressure, slow their heart rate, use less oxygen, and increase relaxed alpha (brain) waves. All of these effects are associated with a lowered metabolic level and with reduced stress. Focusing the mind while relaxing the body may also disrupt harmful psychosomatic patterns, reduce anxiety, reduce muscular tension, improve circulation, restore natural rhythms and balances, and alleviate stress [33]. With so many positive results possible from meditation, you should consider adding the skill to your own repertoire.

Massage

Massage can accomplish a number of things. It can reduce muscle and joint tension, and it can provide the touching or stroking that human beings need, but may not be receiving. Physical massage can be combined with deep breathing and creative visualization. People who tend to be out of touch with their bodies, who need to learn to accept their sensuality, who need nurturing touch, or who need relaxation can benefit from massage [34].

You can give yourself a massage or teach others to do so (Figure 4-15), or learn to give others a massage (Figure 4-16).

Baths

Water can be a powerful relaxant. Fill a bathtub with water that is body temperature. (A thermometer can be hung over the side of the tub.) Immerse yourself up to the neck. This "neutral bath" is so relaxing that "just 15 minutes in this kind of bath is as restful as four hours of sleep" [35].

Humor

Feeling good, and maybe even remaining sane, seems to be related to a sense of humor [36]. Clinicians who work with clients who have problems usually classified as "psychiatric" note that these people do *not* have a sense of humor. In fact, gaining a sense of humor can be a sign that recovery is taking place. Some psychologists, psychiatrists, and mental health nurses have begun to explore the possibilities inherent in humor. Humor has potential as a stress-reduction technique. It is common knowledge that humor can be used to reduce tension in a group; in fact, many speakers use humor to begin their speeches as a way of decreasing audience tension and producing relaxation.

The kind of humor that may be most likely to reduce stress is related to a frame of mind or an attitude toward life [37]. There may be a cluster of qualities that characterize this frame of mind. One is flexibility, or the ability to examine every side of an issue or decision. Another is spontaneity, or the ability to leap from one mode or mood to another with ease. Another is unconventionality, or the ability to free oneself from current values, places, or occupations. Another is shrewdness, or the refusal to believe things or people are what they seem to be. Another is playfulness or the ability to see life as a tragicomic game that can be enjoyed, if not won. Another is humility, or the willingness to question one's importance or the importance of one's achievements, values, or ideas. A final component is irony, or the ability to see that situations are not black and white, that rational actions are often based on irrational feelings, that happy relationships have episodes of suffering and pain, that being humble means having pride, and that truth may change [38]. Figure 4-17 suggests some ways you can enhance your sense of humor.

Dance

Dance therapy allows people to stretch and strengthen muscles and reduce tension. This kind of approach is especially important for those who are inactive because of the work they do or because they have been hospitalized. It is possible to note each individual's area of tension: tight jaw, rigid arms, stiff neck, clenched fists, rigid gait.

Appropriate movement music can be selected, or a small drum or bell can be used to set a rhythm. People who are full of tension or anger can sit on the floor and strike bamboo reeds or sticks on the floor for release. They can also act out daily routines, such as dressing, brushing teeth, or combing hair. People can also do yoga postures or use arm movements derived from folk dances. Swaying the body, interpreting the music, and using props such as scarves, fans, rhythm instruments, balls, and balloons add to the fun and festivity and enhance stress reduction [39].

Music

Music can bring relaxation and emotional refreshment. Music is a nonverbal mode that can be used to release feelings and emotions that have increased their stress level. Music can be listened to or played. Dentists have used soothing background music in their offices for a number of years. Hospitals and clinics should begin to consider the use of classical and/or soothing music. In addition, planned use of music for those under high stress can be initiated in individual hospital rooms, clinic sessions, or wellness programs at home. Music seems to say something to the right hemisphere of our brain—the intuitive, creative side. Clients who have had a stroke or other brain injury can frequently relearn speech if they are sung to, sing back in return, or are spoken to in a rhythmical, emotional way [40].

Poetry

Often, you may be unable to release sufficient tension through movement or verbalizing. In this case, poetry reading/writing can be quite useful. If you are depressed you may be especially able to benefit from this method [41]. Poems can be read you in a one-to-one or a group setting. Poems are chosen for their rhythm, mood or tone, and for the feelings expressed. Discussions about the meaning of the poem can then ensue, and/or you can then write your own poems.

Inner Shouting

Inner shouting is a process where you "spontaneously and without prior thought shout to yourself inside your own head . . ." [42]. Deliberate thinking is discouraged. Instead, blurt out things in a spontaneous way rather than just say or think them quietly. Inner shouting can help you sneak up on the thoughts and feelings you may try to deny, but which increase tension and stress level even when denied. Hurts, pains, or humiliations are focused on; anger is viewed as a symptom, not as the underlying problem. Inner shouting can help you to take responsibility for your feelings of hurt and humiliation. It is useful to start with "shouting" the words, "I feel."

PAIN AND PAIN REDUCTION

Pain is a signal to us that there is something wrong. As such, it is not damaging, but the emotional stress caused by pain can cause physiological damage. Pain is perceived in the brain, so it is responsive to hypnosis, drugs, and suggestions. Touch, voice, and authoritative commands help when people are in acute pain.

There are a number of kinds of pain that are amenable to self-hypnosis. For example, pain due to headache can be treated by suggesting to yourself: "My head will begin to clear in a few minutes, and the excess blood will return to my body. My head is beginning to get less congested, the discomfort is lessening, and soon my headache will be gone." You may have pain for unknown reasons. In these cases, you can suggest to the subconscious that it go to work on the problem, think it over, and realize that for your betterment the condition should be ended [43].

There are other measures that are useful in reducing pain. For example, Dr. David Bresler, director of the UCLA Pain Control Unit, has found that clients who have chronic pain "live in a sea of negativity." For them, he prescribes four hugs a day as an antidote to negativity and as a self-healing measure [44]. If this is a problem of yours you can set a goal of receiving four hugs a day.

People often develop their own ways to deal with pain. Some ways that have been reported as useful are: counting objects; doing mathematical problems; using control phrases ("I won't scream") or supplication phrases ("Hear me"); repeating memorized prayers, rhymes, oaths, or names; evaluating the pain ("It hurts most now" or "The pain is lessening now"); visualizing daily routines such as family discussions or reorganizing a drawer or cupboard; concentrating on lights and shadows; talking to others; pulling or pushing against parts of the body [45].

You can also learn to use a form of self-hypnosis called hypnotic anesthesia to relieve pain; Figure 4–18 gives sample directions for your use [46]. You can use hypnotic anesthesia for childbirth, dental procedures, minor surgery, painful treatments or tests, and so on. The list is endless once you have learned to enhance your innate anesthesia abilities.

Inner dialogue with self is often beneficial for relieving pain. You can learn to direct questions to your inner processes when pain does not abate with other techniques. Sometimes pain continues, because it serves another purpose or because the subconscious misunderstands the need for pain. If you can describe the pain in terms of an animal or an object or like hands pulling or pushing, an inner dialogue can be begun. If you cannot visualize your pain this way, you can get in touch with your inner advisers and then follow the advice you are given. Once you are in touch with the reason for your chronic pain, pain soon moves into a controllable state. (Refer back to Chapter 2 for more information on dialogue with the inner self.)

There are also specific measures you can take for common pains such as back or neck pain. Neck pain can be due to tension (leading to shortening of muscles), weak abdominal muscles (leading to exaggerated low back curve and neck strain), or poor posture while walking, reading, or listening. A test to use to diagnose neck tension is to place the hands in back of the neck at the base of the skull where the muscles meet. If you jump when this spot is pressed, your neck tension is too high and neck pain may soon follow. Some measures to take to decrease the potential for neck pain are [47]:

strengthening abdominal muscles by thinking, "I will hold in my stomach whenever I stand or walk"

correcting gait or posture that may be leading to increased neck stress (this will probably require professional assistance)

losing weight if this is causing undue strain on your abdomen

regularly spending time in a sauna, whirlpool, tub bath, hot shower, or with heating pad on the neck area

standing under a hot shower and slowly moving the neck back and forth; (if a little hurt is noted, continue; if there is a tingling in your arm, stop and see a doctor immediately)

placing chin on chest and then rotating your head in a complete circle in each direction five times a day

doing daily situps (with knees bent, arms across chest, and in a slow manner)

sleeping on a firm mattress

using a chair with an armrest

adjusting your seat for driving or sitting; propping yourself or your reading or work up with pillows so that you do not have to strain to drive, work, or read

washing your hair while standing up in a shower

stretching every hour or two

If you have low back pain you can benefit from specific exercises [48]. One is to lie on your back with knees bent and to press the small of the back against the floor. Another is to lie on your back, grasp hands around your knees, and bring your knees to your chest. Yet another is to bend down on one knee and place both hands flat on the floor at shoulder level; the other leg is extended straight out behind the body, resting on the toes. You can focus on stretching the muscles in the back of the outstretched leg and letting the neck, head, and back relax. This exercise can then be repeated with the other leg outstretched.

ASSERTIVENESS

Assertiveness means the ability to stand up for what "I" feel, think, or desire to do. It means being able to define and stand up for reasonable rights, while being respectful of others' rights. It means being able to set goals for your own wellness, to act on these goals by following through consistently, and to take responsibility for the consequences of your actions. Being assertive requires taking a risk by clearly stating what is expected from others and what they can expect from you.

Aggressive behavior has an element of control or manipulation. "You"-messages such as "Why didn't you . . . ?" "You should have. . . ." and "I think *you* should. . . ." prevail when you are aggressive. A common pattern that develops when you are not assertive is avoidance of a confrontation or wellness issue, build-up of resentment, blow-up or angry outburst, feelings of guilt and recrimination, and a return to avoidance. Thus, aggressiveness/avoidance are intimately connected, and assertive behavior is of a completely different realm. When operating in the assertive realm, issues are addressed, thoughts and feelings are expressed when they occur, and action is taken to enhance wellness.

An especially important part of being assertive is the use of "I" messages. In this case, the speaker takes responsibility for the thought, feeling, or action and does not hedge or blame others. Some "I" messages are: "I feel angry about this." "I think it's time to end this meeting." "I made a mistake." Some "You" (aggressive) messages that *masquerade* as "I" messages are: "I think *you're* wrong." "I feel *you* ought to change." "I want *you* to do as I say." In the first set of messages, the speaker is assertive and does take responsibility for his or her actions, thoughts, and feelings. In the second set of messages, the speaker tries to control the listener by judging his or her behavior, or attempting to force change or action; these messages are really aggressive and avoid the responsibility each person has for his or her behavior.

Some "we" messages can be assertive, especially if they imply collaboration, such as "We can meet and work this out." (Undifferentiated messages, such as, "Let's take our bath now," are *not* assertive *or* collaborative.)

"You" or blaming statements are apt to put others on the defensive; for this reason alone they ought to be deleted. In addition, they attempt to absolve the speaker from his or her responsibility in the issue at hand. Examples of this type of aggressive statement are: "I think this is your fault." "Why didn't you take care of that?" "Why can't *you* do it?" Some assertive statements do use the word *you*—"Would you like to tell me your view?" "I want to thank you."—but there is neither blame nor coercion attached to assertive "you" messages.

People who are unable to express their thoughts and feelings in a direct manner or who feel unappreciated or exploited often report having psychosomatic complaints such as headaches or stomach problems. People who are assertive (or who learn to be so through assertiveness training) frequently report increased feelings of self-confidence, reduced anxiety, decreased bodily complaints, improved communication and response from others [49]. As such, assertiveness can be a stress reduction measure. There are a number of strategies you can use to become more assertive; some of these are discussed below.

Controlling Anxiety, Fear, and Anger

One way to reduce anxiety and fear about being assertive is to learn and regularly practice relaxation exercises. That way you will be prepared to relax totally when you are in situations in which you hope to be assertive. Assertiveness requires the ability to present oneself in a confident, self-assured manner. People whose body musculature is tense and constricted cannot present themselves assertively. A relaxed body increases the probability that clients can approach others in a direct, open way.

Often, people are not aware of how they come across to one another. There are a number of strategies that can be used to provide feedback about presentation of self. Mirror practice can give feedback about facial expression, posture, and whether words fit with gestures and body position. Mirror practice can also be helpful in rehearsing assertive statements prior to trying them with the real-life person. This kind of rehearsal can build confidence so people can present themselves in an assertive way in the upcoming situation.

Audio- and videotape recorders can also provide excellent practice in assertion. Audiotape provides helpful clues about how you sound; whether there are sufficient pauses; whether tone of voice is assertive, aggressive, or avoiding; whether statements are made too quickly; and whether the issue is stated clearly and adhered to. Tape recorders are also useful for recording (and providing instant feedback) regarding your ability to limit interruptions, express feelings appropriately, take a stand on an issue, disagree, admit a mistake, reward or thank another person, give positive criticism, say no, express distress about the way relationships are moving, and ask for collaboration. Some statements to use for practice in these areas are:

I cannot talk to you now. I'll talk to you at one o'clock.

I feel really angry about this!

I have made up my mind on this.

I see your point, but I disagree.

I did make an error.

I appreciate your help.

I think you have demonstrated leadership in this action.

No, I will not reconsider.

I'm upset about our relationship.

Let's sit down and work this out together.

Another use of audiotape is to record relaxing or rewarding messages that can be played back later. For example, Figure 4–4 or 4–5 can be recorded. Some rewarding messages to consider recording are:

You are working toward wellness in a useful, helpful way. Congratulations on your effort. Keep up the good work.

Congratulations on not smoking. Give yourself a hug or find someone to hug. Be proud of yourself. Allow yourself to feel good about yourself.

Videotape feedback adds the extra information of eye contact, body posture and positioning, gestures (especially use of hands), facial expressions, verbal responses that are too quick or hesitant, conciseness of statements, and confidence of presentation. Probably the best use of videotape is in recording upcoming or past situations. Scripts can be written for two or more people and then recorded and evaluated according to each of the information components. Figure 4-19 provides a guide for evaluating an assertive presentation of self.

Another way to use videotape is role playing. In this approach one person tells another person about an upcoming or past situation. The first person gives the other a description of what is to be said, which role each person will take, how the other should act to approximate the real-life situation, and how the interchange will end and begin. Some directions that might apply are: "Be sure to try to make me feel guilty about saying no," or "Every time I try to stick to the issue, you change the subject," or "Use a really angry tone of voice, but pretend you're not angry."

Presentation of self is perhaps the easiest part of assertive behavior. Often, people have deep-seated feelings, thoughts, or beliefs that prevent them from being more assertive. In this case, thought stoppage, examination of counterproductive beliefs, guided fantasy, devising a hierarchy, and structural release of anger can be used. Figures 4-20 to 4-24 give directions for these strategies [50].

Other Assertive Issues

In addition to trying to decrease anxiety, fear, and anger, you may be struggling with issues such as disagreeing with others, limiting others' interruptions on your time, handling a putdown, or asking for legitimate explanations of care. Once you have developed some assertive skills yourself, you can assist others in developing their own skills. The techniques discussed earlier (mirror practice, audio- and videotape replay, role playing, self-evaluation, thought stoppage, examination of counterproductive beliefs, guided fantasy, hierarchies, and structured release of anger) can all be used for this.

SPREADING OUT LIFE CHANGES

Another way of reducing stress is by spreading out life changes and anticipating stressful events. Although there can be little control over unanticipated changes such as accidents or natural disasters, many changes *can* be anticipated and planned for. You may wish to refer back to Figure 3-10, "Changes That May Affect You." Many of these changes can be anticipated and planned for, such as: starting a new school experience, dropping out of school, graduating from school, starting a new job or business, retirement, change in housework status, moving in with someone, moving out, or having someone move in, becoming pregnant, having an abortion, going through menopause, moving, remodeling, taking a vacation, taking out a loan or mortgage, buying a costly item, and holidays. Figure 4-3 can be used to reduce stress.

Thomas H. Holmes is a physician who has studied the effect of life changes on clients' physical health. He has rated life changes in terms of their potential for leading to physical illness. He states that the greater the number of life changes people have during the course of a year, the more likely it is that they will develop a physical illness in the near future [51]. Other researchers disagree [52, 53] and contend that some changes are positive and may not be perceived as stressful, that illness often comes on in a gradual way and is difficult to pinpoint, and that sociocultural values and experiences can lead to differences in what is perceived as stressful. For these (and other reasons) it may be best to treat each change as unique in terms of your stress level. When planning to reduce the potential for life change to lead to illness, the following suggestions may be useful to you:

Become familiar with life events that create change and how these events may affect your life.

Look at Figure 3-10 regularly so you can begin to plan for upcoming changes.

Think about the meaning of expected changes. What will be different as a result of the change? How will you deal with the difference? What assistance from others will you need to deal with the change? How can you rearrange the rest of your life to make this change less stressful for you? Try to identify the feelings you have when you think about the change; do you need help (counseling, teaching, stress reduction skills) from someone else in dealing with the change, or can you use the stress reduction techniques you already know?

Begin to anticipate changes and plan for them well in advance.

Read on your own, or consult with a wellness enhancer about ways to plan for change.

Think about a number of ways (not just one) you can use to adjust to the change.

Use creative visualization, relaxation exercises, self-hypnosis, dialogue with self, centering, thumping your thymus, meditation, massage, baths, humor, dance, music, poetry, and inner shouting to reduce stress related to upcoming change.

Pace changes if you can. For example, try not to move, take on a new job, and get a divorce in the same year, or do a lot of preplanning and anticipatory grief work (see next section) to assist you to reduce your stress level.

GRIEVING FOR LOSSES AND SEPARATIONS

Losing (or gaining) someone or something is always traumatic and results in a time of upheaval. Grief is a normal, expected human reaction. You can provide assistance to yourself or others in identifying losses and separations in actively grieving for them (before, during, and after the loss), and in conveying the idea that grief is an effective way of preventing later illness and loss of optimism about living. One researcher [54] found that a psychological disturbance and a "giving up" syndrome precedes hospitalization for a physical illness. Others [55] found this positive relationship too, but also found changes related to "entrances" (new people) were not as significant as changes related to "exits" (losses). They also noted that society leaves the individual alone to cope with loss, grief, and mourning. Our support systems are more developed around gain than around loss.

The list of losses and separations people can grieve for is very long; some of the more common ones are: loss of teeth; first haircut; amputation of a limb or breast; changes due to accident, illness, or aging; loss of vision, memory, strength, hope, normal elimination route; leaving home; ending a marriage or long-term relationship; loss of a favored pet; changing job or home; loss of friends; death or debilitation of a loved one; graduation from school; change in body shape and feelings during pregnancy or menopause; organ transplant.

The importance of a loss or separation is an individual matter. To some people, the loss of teeth or a favored pet can be just as devastating as surgery or the death of a person.

Originally [56], it was thought that people move through phases of grief, at least in relation to death. Now experts [57] seem to agree that people often experience shock or numbness at the time of a significant loss, but then they tend to move back and forth between denying that there was a loss, being angry and/or depressed that something is being (or has been) lost, coping with the loss by withdrawing, or finding new activities to be interested in. Each person has to be treated as an individual with a specific grief pattern. We do have some information on the reaction of those grieving the loss of a spouse. For example, the widows of men who die from cancer report feeling especially helpless during the illness, while wives of men with chronic heart or blood vessel (cardiovascular) illness felt they were playing an active part in helping their husbands. The widows of men who died from cancer were often angry with nurses and doctors, because they felt that they were abandoned and that their husbands were treated as nonpeople. Some of these widows see their husband's illness as terminal right from the beginning; others see it as a lingering disease where death is not anticipated (despite being told by doctors that their husbands were dying), and death comes as a shock [58].

People who have to learn to accept a significant disability during or after adolescence have an especially hard time finishing with their grief. Just as it seems they are learning to cope, a "trigger experience" can kick off the whole grief process again. Those who become disabled must come face-to-face with their new selves and limitations, with the way their life style is affected, with changes they must make in their life plans, and with learning to live with less than what they counted on. People may learn to live with this kind of a loss, but they may never accept it. With recent technological advances, more and more people will have to learn how to cope with being on a respirator, monitor, kidney machine, or to live with the effects of radical cancer (and other disfiguring) surgeries and near-fatal accidents [59].

It is not only the dying person or surviving spouse who goes through grief. Within a family, various members may be at different stages: some may be denying the loss, others may be angry or depressed [60]. In this case, each person (whether family member or the person with the illness) must be treated as a unique person with a unique grief process.

Examine Figures 4-25 and 4-26 and decide how you might use them in relation to your own or someone else's grief.

SLEEP

It is very difficult to feel well without a good night's sleep. Nutrition, exercise, worry, and tension are some of the variables related to an inability to sleep. To increase your ability to sleep, use the self-hypnosis technique described earlier in this chapter. If you ingest a lot of sugar during the day you may wake up during the night because of a low blood sugar level. There are at least two ways of dealing with this problem: one is to reduce or eliminate sugar intake during the day and increase ingestion of complex carbohydrates. Another is to get up and eat a ripe banana; this will raise the blood sugar level and coax you back to sleep. Warm milk and/or several calcium tablets will also work. Milk contains both calcium that helps to relax muscles, and tryptophane—a precursor of serotonin—a substance related to sleep. If you do not have enough exercise during the day you may have difficulty going to sleep. Some yoga or stretching exercises will help. For the long run, if you have chronic sleep problems you will probably benefit from a daily exercise program. The B-complex vitamins also exert a calming effect and seem to be well tolerated at all doses [61], a vitamin supplement can be considered by clients with sleep problems as it is safer than many sleeping pills that interrupt important sleep/dream patterns, may be addictive, and may have other side effects. Another suggestion is to place a cold cloth on your forehead. This contracts the blood vessels of the head and leads to drowsiness [62].

The neutral or relaxing bath is another method you can use to relax and prepare for sleep. Some herb teas can be used to prepare for sleep. Peppermint, chamomile, or Sleepy Time Tea seem to have a tranquilizing, relaxing effect on the body. Lawrence Gould, a physician, conducted a study to see whether chamomile tea had an adverse effect on people with heart difficulties who had undergone cardiac catheterization. The test showed that drinking the tea had no ill effects, but a hypnotic or sleep-inducing action was noted in 10 of the 12 clients. Cardiac catheterization is a painful, anxiety-provoking procedure [63]. If herb tea can have such a sleep-inducing, tranquilizing effect for these people, think how useful it may be for others. Hot lemonade or grapefruit juice (with or without honey) also seems to be effective. Vickery [64] suggests the following: avoid alcohol, as it disturbs restful sleep; establish a regular bedtime but do not go to bed if wide awake; read (something boring), or listen to soothing music; avoid caffeine (some soft drinks, chocolate, tea, and coffee); have sexual intercourse that is satisfying.

Figure 4-1 /// 167

Figure 4-1   Signs of Need for Relaxation and Stress Reduction

---

Talking signs

talking in an extra-loud, high-pitched voice

finding yourself repeating what you or someone else has already said

spending mealtimes worrying or talking about work or things that bother you

Physical signs

having a "washboard forehead," full of wrinkles

having a tight or sore jaw, face, neck, and/or shoulder area

feeling your head pound as pressures mount

developing headaches, stomach problems, diarrhea, or a spastic colon

feeling tired and dragged out

lying in bed at night with a tense, fixed back

grinding your teeth while sleeping

Worry/approval signs

worrying about the future

having trouble falling asleep due to worry

berating yourself for not doing better

worrying whether others like or approve of you

Time constraints/impatience signs

feeling pressured to get things done

feeling overcommitted

only having time for work

always feeling hurried

feeling that you must attend to the demands of everyone who approaches
you for help

becoming irritated over small, insignificant matters

Leisure/lack of fun signs

reaching for a cigarette, drink, or tranquilizer to feel better

not having any fun any more

always trying to win or compete when playing sports or doing exercises

---

Figure 4-2   Planning to Reduce Stress

Directions:
Answer the questions in Part A. Then go on to Part B and make your plans for reducing your stress level.

PART A

		Yes	No	Some-times

Enjoyment

1.   Every day I focus on enjoying today ....

2.   I eat in a comfortable, leisurely fashion ....

3.   I am able to stand up for my rights and feel good about doing so ....

4.   I take time to separate out trivia from the important, enjoyable things that are the essence of life ....

Time use

5.   I set a time limit on my work, but I don't race the clock ....

6.   I set aside time daily to spend for or with myself ....

7.   I set priorities and don't overload myself with things that aren't important anyway ....

8.   During times of high pressure or responsibllity, I arrange it so someone else can carry some of the load for my usual work ....

9.   I pace my work so I do not end up fighting the clock ....

10.   I can delegate tasks effectively ....

11.   I have time to listen to others' words without interrupting or hurrying them ....

12.   I balance overstimulating situations I am involved in with quiet, restful periods ....

Figure 4–2 /// 169

	Yes	No	Some-times

Attitude

13. I look at rest and relaxation as essential to re-building my reserves, not as "goofing off" ....

14. I try to shrug my shoulders or find the humor in situations rather than clench my teeth or dissolve in anger ....

15. When all around me is in upheaval, I try to view the world as if I'm a detached observer ....

16. I am more interested in the person I am becoming than in the things I am acquiring ....

17. I am convinced that my behavior can increase or decrease my own stress level ....

Self-responsibility

18. I practice the art of smiling at others, conveying warmth and compassion ....

19. I keep a diary of things I react to strongly and then plan how to reduce my reaction to those things ....

20. Several times during each day I relax by using stress-reduction techniques such as meditation or relaxation exercises ....

21. I channel my frustration and anger into con-structive behaviors ....

22. I have at least one hobby or activity that relaxes me ....

23. I am working actively on becoming the person I want to be ....

24. I can admit it to myself and others when I am pushing too hard ....

25. I review my lack of successes to see which were due to impatience and which due to other factors ....

(continued)

Figure 4–2 (continued)

		Yes	No	Some-times
26.	I am willing to take responsibility for reducing my own stress level	......	......	....
27.	I am able to evaluate my strengths and limitations in a neutral way	......	......	....
28.	I plan my life so it is within my limits for change and flexibility	......	......	....
29.	I am working to accept and give criticism and affection with comfort	......	......	....

PART B

1. Look back over your answers. Pay special attention to the statements to which you answered "sometimes" and "no."

2. Choose several areas you want to work on to reduce your stress level. Write down these areas here:

3. Decide on a plan for beginning to work on one or more of these areas, and draw up a contract to that effect.

4. Choose several areas you do *not* want to work on at this time. Write down these areas here:

5. Congratulate yourself on setting priorities and limiting your stress!

Figure 4-3 /// 171

Figure 4-3   Reducing Stressful Life Changes

---

1. Identify your sources of stress by listing changes you have had in the following areas in the past year:

    at school

    at work

    in close relationships with friends, family, and significant other people or pets

    in where or how you live

    in money and finances

    in sudden challenges

    in fears that things will change

2. Look back at your list, and remember how much change or upheaval each change has required or is requiring.

3. Think about changes you will be faced with in the near future.

4. Think about different ways in which you can adjust to each change.

5. List each change and at least two ways you can adjust to each change in the manner shown below:
    upcoming changes   *ways to adjust*

Figure 4-4   Total Body Relaxation Exercise

Step 1:	Ask a friend to read these directions, or record them on tape and play them back.
Step 2:	Lie on a mat on the floor, or sit comfortably in a chair. If possible, remove shoes and restrictive clothing. Choose a quiet, comfortable spot.
Step 3:	Close your eyes, and keep them closed.
Step 4:	Rest your arms comfortably beside you, palms up if you are lying down.
Step 5:	Pull your shoulders down from your ears.
Step 6:	Let your shoulder blades move closer to each other.
Step 7:	Your body is beginning to relax and loosen up now.
Step 8:	Relax your body as you breathe in slowly and deeply from your diaphragm . . . . Let your feet relax . . . . Your feet are more relaxed . . . . Let your ankles relax . . . . Your ankles are relaxing . . . . Let your knees and lower legs relax . . . . Your knees and lower legs are relaxing . . . . Let your thighs relax . . . . Let each layer of muscles of your thighs relax . . . . Let your buttocks relax . . . . Your buttocks or seat is relaxing . . . . Relax your pelvis and groin . . . . Relax . . . . Relax your lower back . . . . Your lower back is relaxing . . . . Relax your diaphragm . . . . Your breathing is becoming easier and more relaxed . . . . Your chest and lungs are relaxing and opening up . . . . Your upper back is relaxing . . . . Relax your shoulders, upper arms, elbows, lower arms, and fingers . . . . Your shoulders and arms are relaxing . . . . Let your neck move easily from side to side . . . . Your neck is relaxing . . . . Relax your head, ears, forehead, eyebrows, eyes, cheeks, and chin . . . . Relax your jaw and chin . . . . Unlock your jaw and relax . . . . Your whole body is relaxing . . . . You feel comfortable, relaxed, peaceful . . . . Continue to relax and enjoy the feeling . . . . When you are ready, slowly open your eyes . . . . Carry this relaxed feeling with you.

Figure 4-5 /// 173

Figure 4-5   Contracting and Relaxing Exercise [7]

Step 1:   Ask someone to read you the directions, or record them on tape and play them back.

Step 2:   Sit comfortably in a chair; loosen your clothing.

Step 3:   Pucker your lips, hold several seconds, relax, and feel the difference. Enjoy the blood flow and relaxation.

Step 4:   Grimace as if you are furious. Hold the grimace several seconds, then relax. Enjoy the feeling.

Step 5:   Squeeze your eyes tightly shut, hold several seconds, then relax your forehead. Enjoy the feeling.

Step 6:   Wrinkle your nose and hold it for several seconds, then release and relax. Enjoy the feeling.

Step 7:   Shut your eyes. Look up as though looking up through the top of your head, then look straight ahead, and relax your eyes. Keep your eyes closed, and look all the way to the right, and then look straight ahead, and relax your eyes. Keep your eyes closed, and look straight ahead, then all the way to the left. Look straight ahead, and relax your eyes. Keep your eyes closed, and look down through your throat, then bring your eyes back to looking straight ahead. Relax your eyes. Move your eyes all around as if following the hands of the clock from 12 to 1 to 2 to 3 to 4 to 5 to 6 to 7 to 8 to 9 to 10 to 11 to 12. Return to looking straight ahead, and relax your eyes. Now follow the hands of your clock from 12 to 11 to 10 and around to 12. Look straight ahead, and then relax your eyes.

Step 8:   Prop your elbows on your knees. Snuggle your relaxed palms over your eyes, being careful not to touch your eyelids. Relax and breathe deeply.

Step 9:   Sit up straight again. Go and get a small glass of cold water. Sit down, and take a small amount of water into your mouth; hold it in your mouth, then swallow, being aware of the coldness as it goes down the back of your throat, down to your stomach. Feel the wave of relaxation as the water goes down.

Step 10:   Sing a high note, and contrast it with a low note. Do this several times, then do it without sound. Then experience the relaxation.

(continued)

Figure 4–5 (continued)

Step 11:   Clench all the muscles in the upper part of your body by pushing the palms of your hands together in front of you. Hold the clench, then relax, and feel the relaxation.

Step 12:   Arch your back, hold the arch, then release, and feel the warmth move down your spine.

Step 13:   Point your toes, and tense all the muscles in your legs; hold, then relax. Feel the relaxation in your legs.

Step 14:   Close your eyes, sit back in your chair, and concentrate on your breathing. Take a deep breath, hold it several seconds, then let it go. Be aware of the relaxation as you let it go.

Step 15:   Keeping your eyes closed, scan your body for tense muscle groups. Breathe in, hold it, then breathe out, saying "Relax" as you relax those muscles. Note any tension, tense that spot even more, then let it go. Each time, think of the word, "Relax" when breathing out. Continue until all of you is relaxed.

Keep practicing daily until you can relax by merely saying the word, "Relax." When you feel very tense, repeat steps 1 through 15.

Figure 4-6 /// 175

Figure 4-6   Relaxing Tense Facial Muscles

Step 1:   Go to a quiet, relaxing spot.

Step 2:   Close your eyes, inhale deeply, and exhale as you slowly and gently press your thumbs above your collarbone while pressing your fingers against your upper shoulder blade areas. Hold the position for two minutes while breathing comfortably, then relax. Allow yourself to feel your face relaxing.

Step 3:   Lie down on a rug, mat, or bed. Lace your fingers loosely together, making a cradle for the middle of the back of your head. Press your thumbs against the base of your skull. Inhale deeply, press your thumb, then exhale. Continue to press, inhale, and exhale for two minutes, then drop your hands to your sides, and relax. Allow your face to relax.

Step 4:   Slowly sit up, and press your thumbs gently into the spot where your jaw hinges (in front of your ears); place your fingertips lightly on your forehead. Breathe comfortably, holding the position for two minutes.

Step 5:   Lie down with your eyes closed, and enjoy peace and relaxation.

Figure 4-7 Relaxing Stiff Back and Shoulders [8]

Step 1:   Sit in a straight-backed chair and cross your legs, with the left knee on top. Hold on to the left knee with the right hand. Hold the knee in place and look as far as you can over the *right* shoulder. Do this in a slow, controlled movement. Be sure not to strain. Breathe in and out comfortably as you stretch. Then repeat on the other side (recrossing your legs the other way).

Step 2:   Lie on your stomach, but hold your head and chest up with your arms stretched out in front of you. Twist your head slowly to one side, trying to look at your heel. Do *not* force; turn in an easy, controlled stretch. Return your head to the front, and then twist to the other side.

Step 3:   Support yourself by holding onto a chair with one hand. Bend your body forward at the waist. Allow your other arm to swing easily at your side. Swing this arm from side to side and back and forth and then in a clockwise and counterclockwise fashion. Repeat, using the other arm.

Step 4:   Get down on the floor on your hands and knees, with your hands quite a bit forward. Keep elbows stiff while bringing your hips down toward your heels in a slow, controlled stretch. Hold a few seconds, then relax.

For people who have already developed pain or infliction, these exercises should be done *very* gently. For those who sit all day at work or home, the exercises serve as a preventive measure against immobility; in this case the exercises can be done with more vigor.

Figure 4-8 /// 177

Figure 4-8   Releasing Shoulder and Neck Tension

Step 1:   Stand up, clasp hands behind back, keeping elbows straight, palms touching. Roll your elbows in trying to touch your elbows together. Hold in a controlled stretch. Release hands, and let them go to a comfortable spot alongside your body.

Step 2:   Cup your right hand, and slap your left shoulder muscle about ten times. Cup your left hand, and slap your right shoulder muscle about ten times. Put your hands at your sides, and bring your shoulders up to ears and back down again. Circle one shoulder, then the other, then both. Write your name with each shoulder. Sway your body to the right and then to the left. Make believe you are a young tree bending in the wind. Let your body relax.

Step 3:   Sit on the floor. Wrap your arms around your knees and around your back. Make yourself as small as possible. Bring your heels close to your thigh muscles. Pretend you are a small ball. Tighten the muscles in your face, eyes, and mouth. Hold this position for 15 seconds. Then release, lie down with your feet comfortably apart and your arms overhead. Stretch your fingers and toes. Open your mouth, stick your tongue out, and open your eyes as wide as you can. Then relax your body, and feel the energy and relaxation flowing to all parts of your body. Let your body float in relaxation.

Figure 4-9   Relax Your Feet, Relax Your Body [9]

These exercises can be used by persons who are in bed or who sit up all day. They can also be used for relaxation after vigorous exercise or stressful situations, for energizing oneself.

Step 1:   *Look* at your bare feet. Ask yourself, "What can I feel in my feet?" See what each foot looks like.

Step 2:   Take each toe on one foot, and gently rotate it in a small circle. Roll each toe between your thumb and index finger.

Step 3:   Easily massage the pads of your foot. Push firmly against your toenails.

Step 4:   Pull at each toe gently. Place your thumb behind each joint, and push slightly.

Step 5:   Massage the ball of your foot firmly.

Step 6:   Use your thumb to press down the outside of the arch, over the surface of the heel, up the other side of your foot, and up the Achilles tendon above your heel.

Step 7:   Ask yourself now, "How does my foot feel now?" "How does the rest of my body feel?"

Step 8:   Do the same exercise with the other foot.

Figure 4–10 /// 179

Figure 4–10   Alternate-Nostril Breathing [10,11]

Step 1:   Rest your right thumb lightly against your right nostril. Rest your ring and little finger lightly against your left nostril. Exhale slowly and deeply through both nostrils.

Step 2:   Press your right nostril closed with your right thumb. Slowly inhale, taking a deep breath through your left nostril, counting to four as you inhale.

Step 3:   Open your right nostril, and exhale through it to a rhythmic count of four.

Step 4:   Without pausing, inhale through your right nostril to a rhythmic count of four.

Step 5:   Open your left nostril, and exhale through it for four counts.

Steps 1 through 5 makes up a round.

Repeat this cycle for 5 or 10 rounds. Take care to keep your breathing slow and even.

As you become skilled in this exercise, you can begin to hold your breath for four counts between inhaling and exhaling.

Figure 4–11   Reducing Tension at Home or at Work

Exercise 1,   *releasing tension while talking on the phone:*

Circle your shoulder, switch the receiver to the other ear, circle your shoulder. Try to touch your shoulder blades together in back, and then try to touch your shoulders together in front. Every time you reach for the phone, circle your shoulders. Place your hand on your hip, stand up, and circle the upper part of your body around as you talk. Place your other hand on your other hip and repeat.

Exercise 2,   *releasing tension in your lower back:*

While sitting in a chair, inhale deeply, and press your back against the back of the chair. Hold for 10 seconds, then release your back from the chair, exhale, and let all the tension flow out of your body.

Exercise 3,   *releasing tension in legs and arms:*

While sitting in a chair, raise your legs, and make several circles with your ankles; reverse the circle. Put your feet back on the floor, and observe the effect. Now make several circles with your wrists in each direction. Make several circles with your arms in each direction. Let your arms drop slowly to your sides. Relax your legs and arms deeply.

Exercise 4,   *releasing tension in neck:*

Roll your head easily over to your left shoulder, let your head dangle on your neck, and fall back. Slowly rotate your head over to your right shoulder. Pretend your head is bobbing loosely on your shoulders. Let your head bob from your right shoulder to your chest. Slowly rotate your head around in this manner until your neck relaxes. Now rotate your head around in the other direction until you feel deep relaxation in your neck.

Figure 4–12 /// 181

Figure 4–12   Directions for Self-Hypnosis

Step 1: Write out in detail *exactly* what you hope to accomplish. Now condense the idea into one or two sentences. Be sure to use positive suggestion.

Step 2: Ask someone to read the following directions or record them on tape until you are familiar with what to do.

Step 3: Sit or lie down in a comfortable position.

Step 4: Choose a fixed object to focus on: a picture on the wall, a spot on the ceiling, a fire in the fireplace, or a lighted candle.

Step 5: Watch the fixed object intently.

Step 6: Do some alternate-nostril breathing (Figure 4–9) while watching the fixed object.

Step 7: Give yourself a suggestion that you will awake after a certain amount of minutes, or at a specific time.

Step 8: Think only about your breathing, and watch the fixed object. Give yourself the following suggestion: "As I watch this candle (flame, object) my eyelids will become heavier and heavier. Soon they will be so heavy they will close. Soon I will be in hypnosis." Use your own words, and repeat the suggestion until your eyelids begin to feel heavy. Let them close when you are ready.

Step 9: As your eyes close, use a key word or phrase to signal your subconscious to bring you to hypnosis; for example, repeat the words, "relax now" slowly three times.

Step 10: Begin to relax your body. Start at your feet . . . . Relax your toes, . . . your ankles, . . . your calves, . . . your knees, . . . your thighs. . . . Let your legs go limp . . . . Let your stomach and abdominal muscles relax . . . . You are letting go, . . . feeling more and more relaxed . . . . Let your chest and breathing muscles relax . . . . You are starting to breathe more easily from the lower part of your lungs . . . . Your breathing and pulse are gradually slowing down, . . . slowing down, . . . Sinking deeper, . . . sinking deeper into relaxation . . . . Let your back muscles relax, . . . your back muscles are relaxing . . . . Your shoulders, . . . upper arms, . . . elbows, . . . lower arms, . . . and fingers are relaxing . . . . As you go deeper, your face is relaxing . . . . Let your face relax.

Step 11: Think to yourself, "Now I am going deeper and deeper." Repeat this thought several times.

(continued)

Figure 4–12 (continued)

Step 12:   Unless you dislike riding escalators,* imagine yourself standing at the top of one. Feel yourself going down, down, down on the escalator. Count backwards slowly from ten to zero, imagining you are going down on the escalator. (Take yourself down three floors this way until you become more proficient; at that point, one floor will do.)

Step 13:   When you wish to awaken yourself, think, "Now I am going to wake up."

Step 14:   Give yourself the suggestion, "When I awake, I will feel relaxed and refreshed; I will carry this feeling with me throughout my day."

Step 15:   Slowly count backward from five to one, and slowly open your eyes.

*Substitute an elevator or staircase; you may also ride or walk up—in this case substitute the word, farther for deeper.

Figure 4-13 /// *183*

Figure 4-13   Going to a Peaceful Spot in your Mind: Creative Visualization

Close your eyes, now . . . . Listen to the sound of my voice . . . . I am going to
take you on a trip to the mountains . . . . You get into your van and think of the
peaceful relaxing mountains . . . . Your van begins to move, and you are enjoying the easy sway of the van . . . . The windows are open, and you can feel
the warm sun and the cool breeze . . . . You are beginning to relax and unwind
. . . . The van begins to go up, up, up the mountain . . . . Winding slowly and
easily up the mountain . . . . You are relaxing, smelling the flowers, hearing the
birds chirp, feeling the warm sun, seeing the blue sky and white clouds . . . . The
van pulls up beside a lake at the foot of the mountain . . . . You move easily to
the lake . . . . You watch the ripples in the lake, feel the cool breeze on your
face and the warm sun on your face, arms, and hands . . . . You look up at the
mountain, see the snow on top, and feel more and more relaxed and peaceful
. . . . You watch several ducks float across the lake, leaving ripples in the water
behind them . . . . You watch the ripples, feeling more and more relaxed and
comfortable . . . . Now I am going to be quiet for a few minutes and let you
stay at the mountains, getting more and more relaxed as each moment
passes . . . . (Pause for several minutes, letting yourself relax.) . . . . Now I'm
going to take you back from the mountains, and you're going to bring that relaxed and peaceful feeling with you . . . . Whenever you want return to that
feeling and that place, just close your eyes and think of the word SIGMA,
SIGMA, and you will feel relaxed and peaceful . . . . I will count back from five,
and when I reach one, you will open your eyes and feel relaxed and refreshed
. . . . Five, . . . four, . . . three, . . . two, . . . one . . . . (Pause.) . . . . Tell me
what you experienced while you were at the mountains.

Figure 4–14   Directions for Meditation

Step 1:   Find a quiet, comfortable room. Take the phone off the hook, close the door, and let family members know you are meditating. If at work, place a sign on your door.

Step 2:   Sit in a straight-backed chair or on the floor.

Step 3:   Imagine your spine becoming longer and more elastic.

Step 4:   Assume there is a silken cord attached to the top of your head, exerting a slight pull upward, expanding your chest cavity and pulling your rib cage up out of your abdominal cavity, giving you more space to breathe easily.

Step 5:   Close your eyes, and keep them closed.

Step 6:   Visualize yourself enveloped in a golden, soothing circle of warmth.

Step 7:   Focus your awareness on your heart, on the left side of your chest. Breathe in and out in a relaxed way, expanding your chest cavity as you take in air.

Step 8:   Breathe in as if your heart were a mouth that fills you with golden warmth and light. Allow yourself to feel your whole body filling up with this warmth and light. Breathe deeply and slowly, imagining your heart as open to receive the light and warmth. As you exhale, let out all doubts, anger, fear, sadness, thoughts, illness, imbalance, and anything that prevents you from feeling at peace with yourself.

Step 9:   Continue to breathe in warmth and light and breathe out troublesome feelings, thoughts, imbalances.

Step 10:   Pay no attention to thoughts. Concentrate on your breathing for 20 to 30 minutes.

Be sure to meditate every day.

Figure 4-15 /// 185

Figure 4-15   Directions for a Self-Massage

Step 1:   Move your fingers vigorously in a circular movement and in a caressing, loving way, while breathing deeply and easily. Follow the route that appears below.

Step 2:   Gently massage your head and hair. Massage the back of your head to the base of your skull. Massage the top, side, and back of your ears.

Step 3:   Caress and massage your forehead. Massage your cheeks lightly.

Step 4:   Stroke firmly up your throat to your chin. Use a circular massage motion with your fingertips all around the back of your neck.

Step 5:   Use your right hand to knead and massage your left shoulder and down your left arm. Knead your left thumb, each one of your fingers on your left hand, and the palm and top of your left hand.

Step 6:   Use your left hand to knead and massage your right shoulder and down your right arm. Knead your right thumb, each one of your fingers on your right hand, and the palm and top of your right hand.

Step 7:   Use your left or right hand to massage your chest and abdomen.

Step 8:   Use both your hands to massage as much of your back and buttocks as possible.

Step 9:   Move your hands to the upper part of your left thigh. Use both hands to massage down your leg. Sit down, and massage your feet. (Refer to Figure 4-9.)

Step 10:   Stand up, and use both hands to massage your right leg.

Step 11:   Observe the effect of your caressing, loving touch.

(Optional step): Either before or after your massage, use a loofah sponge to bring healing energy and blood to your back, legs, and arms.

Figure 4-16   Directions for Giving a Massage to Another Person

---

General Directions:

Keep your hands flexible and relaxed. Use your hands to fit the contours of the client's body. Experiment with different strokes, speeds, and pressures. Ask the other person for feedback about your technique. Try to relax and enjoy the experience.

Step 1:   Choose a warm, comfortable room. Ask the person to remove all clothes and lie face down on a padded floor on an old sheet. If the client is cold or modest, he or she can be covered during the massage in any area not being massaged.

Step 2:   Kneel down beside the other person. Place some massage or vegetable oil in your hands, and rub them together until the oil feels warm.

Step 3:   Ask the person to relax and breathe easily. Tell him or her to anticipate a relaxing massage.

Step 4:   Maintain contact with the person's body during the massage. If you need more oil, rest one hand on his or her back and pour oil into it. Place your hands on the shoulder blades. Slowly and firmly slide up to the shoulders, over the top of the arms, back down the shoulders, down the buttocks, let the palms slide gently up each side of the spine, and repeat the cycle until the back becomes more relaxed to the touch.

Step 5:   Place your right hand, faced in, across the left ankle. Place your left hand above the right hand, facing out. Glide both hands to the top of the leg, moving lightly over the knee. Repeat on the right leg.

Step 6:   Ask the person to use one finger of the right hand to indicate she or he is ready to turn over and two fingers if more massage is needed.

Step 7:   When the person is ready to turn over, place your hands around the right arm and glide the hands firmly down the arm to the elbow and then down to the wrist. Squeeze the fleshy parts of the hand, and pull and squeeze the fingers. Repeat with the left arm.

Step 8:   Move down the left thigh to the ankle. Squeeze the fleshy parts of the foot; pull and squeeze the toes. Repeat with the right thigh and leg.

Figure 4-17 /// 187

Figure 4-17   Activities to Use to Develop a Sense of Humor

Directions:

Using the seven components of humor (flexibility, spontaneity, unconvention-ality, shrewdness, playfulness, humility, and irony) practice ways of enhancing your sense of humor, and of seeing your problems in a humorous way.

Flexibility

1.   Look at the situation from many different points of view, for example, from a child's, parent's, spouse's, boss', religious person's, doctor's, nurse's, or alien-visitor-from-another-planet's point of view.

2.   Be your problem, and ask, "What kind of clothes would my problem wear?" "What language would it talk?" "What songs would it sing?" "What mottos would it have?"

3.   Make a list of dreams, hunches, fantasies, wild ideas, or wishes you have had. Review the list and see how it bears on your level of wellness.

Spontaneity

1.   Decide how to solve a problem using intellectual or logical processes. Then solve the same problem using your intuitive or feeling reactions. Next, solve the same problem using a spiritual or cosmic approach.

2.   Demonstrate different feelings through using facial expression, body posture, and any other mode but words. Some feelings to use are: anger, love, sadness, fear.

Unconventionality

1.   Plan a day in your life as if you were living in a Kibbutz in Israel, an Indian reservation, an Eskimo village, a spaceship circling the moon, and Krypton (Superman's birthplace).

2.   Live one day as if you were Louis Pasteur, Florence Nightingale, Madame Curie, Wonder Woman, Albert Einstein, a favorite animal or bird.

Shrewdness

1.   Give examples of how you are not who you seem to be.

2.   Think about your friends, family, and other significant people. Draw up a list of people, and then write down at least one example of how each person is not who he or she seems to be.

(continued)

Figure 4–17 (continued)

Playfulness

1. Pretend your current predicament is a game. Write down the rules and chance factors that are operating, draw up game cards, a score sheet, and rules for who wins and loses.
2. Visualize your total life as a game. Chart "wins," "losses," and "rained out" events. List times of enjoyment, fun, sadness, and fear. Give a name to your life game.

Humility

1. State the meaning of life for you. Consider what would happen if that were *not* the meaning of life.
2. Pretend you are an ant or a mosquito. Try to expand on what your life would be like.

Irony

1. Think about how ironic life is, and to try to remember how happy events or relationships have included suffering, and difficult situations have brought happiness.
2. List your greatest desires or fears at the moment. Then look at the list and ask for each entry, "What difference does this make in terms of my total life or of the larger scheme of eternity?"

Figure 4-18 /// 189

Figure 4-18   Directions for Inducing Hypnotic Anesthesia [46]

Step 1:   Become completely relaxed and in a hypnotic state.

Step 2:   (Refer to Figure 4-12.) Clear your mind of any doubts about being able to anesthetize yourself.

Step 3:   With your eyes closed, imagine there is a row of electric light switches in your head. Each switch has a light above it of a different color, and each goes to a different part of your body. The switch with the blue light above it goes to your right hand. Assure yourself that you *can* do this task.

Step 4:   Imagine you are turning on the blue light now.

Step 5:   Repeat the following suggestions several times each:
"My hand is getting more and more numb and may feel slightly cooler." Allow yourself to be confident about this task.

Step 6:   In a minute or so, say "In a minute I am going to pinch my right hand, and it will be anesthetized so all I will feel is pressure. It will be as if I am pinching a thin leather glove. Af first I will pinch lightly. Each time I pinch, the anesthesia will increase. When I have pinched five times, my right hand will be anesthetized."

Step 7:   Continue to pinch the right hand at short intervals, increasing the strength of the pinch each time, realizing that you will feel only pressure each time you pinch. Be aware that the first time you complete this practice session your hand may be only partially anesthetized, but by pinching your other hand, you *will* notice a difference between them.

Step 8:   *Always remember to remove the anesthesia* when it has served its purpose by using the thought, "My right hand (or whatever body part you are using) will be as it was before, and I will be able to feel everything I could before anesthesia."

Step 9:   Continue to practice the technique until you can anesthetize your hand by saying, "When I stroke my right hand three times I will feel only pressure when I pinch it."

Step 10:   Practice learning to shut off pain to other body parts until you can induce anesthesia at will.

Figure 4-19   Evaluate Your Own Assertiveness

Directions:

Rate yourself in each category; practice on the categories you were not pleased with in terms of your performance.

		I was pleased	*I need to practice this*

1. *Nonverbal presentation*

    a.   eye contact

    b.   relaxed posture

    c.   nervous laughter

    d.   joking

    e.   excessive or contradictory gestures

    f.   low level of anxiety

2. *Verbal content*

    a.   communicated what was intended

    b.   spoke concisely and clearly

    c.   stuck to the point

    d.   apologetic comments

    e.   overly long explanations

    f.   used "I" or "we-collaborative" statements

3 *Verbal presentation*

    a.   spoke too quickly or too slowly

    b.   stammered

    c.   hesitated

    d.   too loud or too soft

    e.   whined

    f.   pleaded

    g.   was sarcastic

Figure 4-20 /// *191*

Figure 4-20   Directions for Decreasing Self-Anger through Thought Stoppage

---

Step 1:   List self-defeating or angry-at-self thoughts you have. If you are having trouble identifying this kind of thought, read the statements that follow; these are thoughts that have been used by others: "I can't be assertive." "Assertiveness just won't work." "I'm stupid." "I'll never learn this."

Step 2:   Choose one self-defeating thought.

Step 3:   When the thought begins to form in your mind, say, loudly and clearly, "Stop!" Continue to say "stop!" more loudly and clearly until the thought recedes.

Step 4:   When you are able to stop the thought at will, consciously ask yourself to have the thought. When the thought begins to form, say, "Stop!" in a loud and clear manner. When the thought stops, say, "Relax" and allow yourself to feel calm and relaxed.

Step 5:   Continue to practice Step 4 until you can conjure up the thought, make it recede, and relax.

Step 6:   Practice mastering thought stoppage by merely *thinking* the word "Stop!" Conjure up the thought, "*Think* Stop!" and concentrate on the word. When the thought stops, say "Relax," and allow yourself to feel calm and relaxed.

Step 7:   Choose another self-defeating thought and practice Steps 1 through 6.

Be aware that at first, your self-defeating thoughts may increase in number. Continue to practice as this is an expected happening when you focus in on them. As you practice, your skill in stopping self-defeating thoughts will increase, and the frequency of this kind of thought will decrease, so persevere!

Figure 4–21 Examining Counterproductive Beliefs that Inhibit Assertiveness

---

Directions:

You may need to examine your counterproductive beliefs about being assertive if you notice the following cues: You are not becoming more assertive despite practice, and if you continue to be uncomfortable when practicing, continue to stumble or falter in your speech despite knowing what to say, or continue to be aggressive or fear that you won't be able to cope despite knowing assertiveness is appropriate. If you notice one or more of these cues, examine your counterproductive beliefs, using the steps below:

Step 1: Ask yourself, what belief or attitude do I hold that is keeping me from being more assertive? If you have difficulty identifying your counterproductive beliefs, read through the list that follows and see if you hold any of them:

It's not right to disagree with others, especially those in authority.

I do not have the right to express my thoughts or feelings directly.

I am responsible for other people's feelings or reactions.

I am not permitted to make a mistake.

I should never say no to a request.

I can't change the way things are.

I should always be understanding.

I should be able to handle whatever workload I am asked to do.

If I take a risk and act assertively, it may prove fatal.

Step 2: Begin to challenge one of your counterproductive beliefs by asking the following questions:

Why do I think this belief is true?

If I learned this belief earlier in my life, does it still hold true now?

Do I want to continue to hold this belief even though it may not make me feel good about myself?

Is it good for my health (blood pressure, stress level, etc.) to hold this belief?

Does holding this belief deny my rights as a person?

Does this belief seem overprotective of myself and others?

Figure 4-21 /// 193

If I were the other person in an assertive interchange, would *I* be devastated by one act of assertiveness?

If other people are responsible for their own feelings and actions, can my being assertive hurt them?

Step 3:   If you find Step 2 difficult, find a friend or family member who can help you question your beliefs. Pick a person who does not hold the same counterproductive beliefs you do.

Figure 4–22   Using Guided Fantasy to Increase Assertiveness

Step 1:   Think of a two-person situation in which you want to be assertive. Picture every detail of the situation: who is there with you, where the incident takes place, and what the interchange is about.

Step 2:   Remember that you are the creator of this experience. You can make happen whatever you want in the private screening room in your mind.

Step 3:   Close your eyes and begin to see yourself being assertive in the situation you chose. Write yourself a mental script, and coach yourself about your posture, gestures, and tone of voice so you sound and look assertive. Keep the other person in the situation on hold, as if he or she is frozen in a listening attitude. Go on with your assertive speech, paying close attention to the details of your presentation. If you are not completely satisfied with your performance, redo it while keeping the other person frozen in a listening attitude.

Step 4:   When you have completed your assertive performance in a way that feels good to you, congratulate yourself on your assertiveness. Allow yourself to feel good about what you said or did.

Step 5:   When you have mastered your presentation of self, imagine the other person now being able to respond to your assertiveness. Imagine watching his or her response as if you are in a theater watching a movie. You are detached and able to view his or her response as if from a distance; you remain confident in your right to express yourself regardless of how the other person reacts. You are able to remain calm and convinced about your point of view. If you picture the other person as assertive, too, you may decide to collaborate with him or her. If not, be sure to picture yourself sticking to the issue and not becoming sidetracked by unrelated arguments, attempts to make you feel guilty or intimidated, nagging, procrastination, or unfair criticism. Practice this part of your guided fantasy until you feel comfortable with your reactions. If you become anxious or fearful, stop your practice and complete a relaxation exercise, then return to your practice.

Step 6:   When you have completed your guided fantasy to your satisfaction, congratulate yourself on your accomplishment.

Step 7:   Decide how you will implement what you learned from your guided fantasy practice.

Figure 4-23 /// 195

Figure 4-23   Devising a Hierarchy to Learn Assertive Behavior

---

Directions:

Use this exercise if you are anxious of fearful about an upcoming situation and want gradual practice in overcoming your anxiety or fear.

Step 1:   Choose an upcoming situation about which you feel anxious or fearful.

Step 2:   Break the situation down into its components. For example, if you are anxious about asking your boss for a raise, you might break this down into the following steps:

1.   waking up the day you will ask your boss for a raise

2.   remembering you have an appointment to talk with your boss

3.   driving to work and thinking about the upcoming meeting

4.   arriving at work, looking at your calendar, and seeing the appointment schedule

5.   noticing it is time to go to your appointment

6.   sitting outside his or her office

7.   entering his or her office

8.   beginning to speak with your boss

9.   asking your boss for a raise

Step 3:   Once you have broken your situation down into its component parts, number the least anxiety-provoking as number 1, and the most anxiety-provoking with the highest number.

Step 4:   Now think about being in the situation described in number 1. Visualize the situation in your mind. If you find yourself becoming anxious, do a relaxation exercise (refer to Chapter 3), then return to visualizing the situation, until you feel relaxed while visualizing it.

Step 5:   Move on through the rest of the steps, stopping to use a relaxation exercise until you are comfortable visualizing each step.

Step 6:   Plan when you will implement your assertive behavior in real life.

Step 7:   On the day you choose to practice your new assertive behavior, use relaxation exercises at each step toward your goal. Reward yourself when you meet your goal.

Figure 4–24   Releasing Anger in a Structured Way

Directions:

Use this exercise when you believe it is unwise to express your anger directly with another person or when you have tried to do so and been retaliated against for being assertive. In other words, this kind of exercise is useful when direct assertiveness does not give you satisfaction, and you need an outlet for your anger.

Step 1:   Imagine the situation in which you were furious about how you were treated. Conjure up the angry feeling and allow yourself to experience it to the fullest. Be aware that it is O.K. to be angry and that you *can* find a constructive outlet for it.

Step 2:   Pretend you are running a movie in your mind where you, as director, are able to change the actual events and make them turn out as you wish. Allow yourself to feel power and mastery over the situation. Pretend you are both actor and director in this movie. Coach yourself to say or do what you wish you could have done in the real-life situation. Use your full creative powers to show how angry you are. You may decide to use physical aggression in your movie; remind yourself this is O.K. to do since it is not hurting anyone, and it is only a fantasy you are directing and controlling.

Step 3:   If you still feel angry, find a pillow and a quiet place. Imagine that the pillow is the person with whom you are angry. Punch that pillow while releasing all your anger through the punching and through shouting out loud all the anger and hurt you feel. Continue in this manner until you feel you have released your anger and loosened yourself from the control this situation had over you.

Step 4:   Allow yourself to feel good about dealing with your anger in a structural, constructive way. Believe that you can now stand back from the situation, view its humorous aspects, and have a sense of detachment from it.

Figure 4-25 /// 197

Figure 4–25   Using Creative Visualization to Separate from Someone

---

Directions:

This exercise can be used to assist you through a separation/grief process. Adapt it to fit each unique person.

Step 1:   Allow yourself to relax completely. Use one of the relaxation exercises described in Chapter 3.

Step 2:   Imagine yourself sitting with the person from whom you are separating. Imagine everything about that person and your relationship with him or her. Allow yourself to see the strengths and weaknesses of this person, to recount your relationship with this person in a step-by-step manner. Allow yourself to experience the highs and lows of the relationship. Visualize yourself bound to the person by thin but strong silken ties, each representing a facet of your relationship.

Step 3:   Once you have visualized all aspects of your relationship and are able to see and feel the ties that bind you together, imagine the ties loosening one by one. Imagine yourself as being freed from the relationship while at the same time taking with you positive feelings about what you were able to give to one another while the relationship lasted. Now feel yourself beginning to loosen your ties to this person, see yourself rise from your seat, give this person a final good-bye, and leave, feeling free and happy and glad that you were able to have had this experience in your lifetime. See yourself moving onto a new path, a path full of light, energy, and interest. Know that although this relationship is ending, it will give you strength and knowledge to build new ones. Allow yourself to experience the strength and revelation of this moment. Carry these pictures and feelings with you as you set out to find a new life for yourself. Allow yourself to realize that you can create new loving relationships for yourself.

Figure 4–26 Imagining Happiness for a Grief-Stricken Person in Your Life

---

Directions:

Family members or friends often ask what they can do to help people who are grieving. This exercise can be done to transfer positive energy from friends or family to the grief-stricken person.

Step 1:   Use one of the relaxation exercises described in Chapter 3 to relax and center yourself; become attuned to your inner processes and your place in the universe.

Step 2:   Picture in your mind's eye that grieving person you are concerned about. Take yourself back to happier times when he or she seemed strong and confident. You now have two pictures of the person in your mind, a split-screen effect. Now picture pouring energy from the figure representing happier times over to the grief-stricken figure. Imagine that the more energy you pour, the stronger and more confident each image becomes. Realize that there is infinite energy available to you and to this person about whom you are concerned. Picture the energy flowing into this person as if a bright light is encasing him or her and providing renewal and strength. Carry this new image of this grieving person with you. Bear in mind that you can be helpful to this person through your positive, energy-giving visualizations. Be sure to visualize this image when you are with the person you are concerned about.

NOTES

1. Hans Selye. *Stress without Distress*. New York: Lippincott, 1974, p. 111.
2. Ibid., pp. 14, 18.
3. Herbert Benson. *The Relaxation Response*. New York: Avon, 1975, p. 29.
4. Meyer Freidman and Ray Rosenman. *Type A Behavior and Your Heart*, New York: Alfred A. Knopf, 1974, p. 4.
5. Kathy Slobogin. "Stress," *New York Times Magazine* (November 20, 1977), pp. 48-106.
6. Ibid., p. 50.
7. Based on Dr. James Ferguson. "Deep muscle relaxation," The Health Field, NBC, March 11, 1979.
8. Chester E. Kirk. "Loosen up your tight, aching shoulders," *Prevention* (April 1977), pp. 70-76.
9. Lilias. Yoga, and You, Channel 13, March 13, 1979.
10. Lorin Pepper. "Alternate nostril breathing." In *The Holistic Health Handbook*, by Ed Bauman, Armand Ian Brint, Lorin Print, and Pamela Amelia Wright, Berkeley, Calif.: And/Or Press, 1978, p. 43.
11. Jess Stearn. *Yoga, Youth and Reincarnation*. New York: Bantam, 1965, pp. 319-320.
12. Roger Bernhardt and David Martin. *Self-Mastery Through Self-Hypnosis*. New York: Signet, 1977, pp. 1-17.
13. Leslie M. LeCron. *Self Hypnotism: The Technique and Its Use in Daily Living*. New York: Signet, 1964, p. 42.
14. Bernhardt and Martin, *Self-Mastery*, pp. 19-20.
15. LeCron, *Self Hypnotism*, pp. 44-45.
16. Ibid., pp. 25, 78-80.
17. Ibid., pp. 86-92.
18. Bernhardt and Martin, *Self-Mastery*, p. 1.
19. Ibid., pp. 9-10.
20. LeCron, *Self Hypnotism*, pp. 49-62.
21. Bernhardt and Martin, *Self-Mastery*, pp. 63-64.
22. Ibid., pp. 60-74.
23. LeCron, *Self Hypnotism*, p. 65.
24. Bernhardt and Martin, *Self-Mastery*, pp. 64-68.
25. Joannie Porter. "Suggestions and success imagery for study problems," *The International Journal of Clinical and Experimental Hypnosis* 26, no. 2 (1978), pp. 63-75.
26. John Diamond. *BK Behavioral Kinesiology*. New York: Harper & Row, 1979, p. 31.
27. Ibid., p. 33.
28. Ibid., p. 37.
29. Ibid., pp. 39, 43-44, 49, 63, 99.
30. Ibid., p. 122.
31. Ibid., p. 35.

32. Ibid., pp. 41–44, 62, 66, 100–101, 119–122.
33. Kathleen Riordon Speeth. "The healing potential of meditation." In Bauman et al., *Holistic Health*, pp. 246–253.
34. Margaret Elke and Mel Resinan. "Sensitive massage." In Bauman et al., *Holistic Health*, pp. 175–179.
35. "My two techniques for eliminating nervous tension," *The Health Newsletter* no. 16 (1978), p. 5.
36. Harvey Mindess. "The sense in humor," *Saturday Review* (August 21, 1971), pp. 10–12.
37. Ibid.
38. Don Koberg and Jim Bagnall. *The Universal Traveler.* Los Altos, Calif.: William Kaufman, 1973, p. 40.
39. Esther C. Frankel. "Dance therapy." In *The Practical Encyclopedia of Natural Healing* by Mark Bricklin. Emmaus, Pa.: Rodale, 1976, pp. 120–128.
40. Laurel Elizabeth Keyes. *Toning: The Creative Power of the Voice.* De Vorss Pub., 1973.
41. Judith C. Wood. "Poetry therapy," *Journal of Psychiatric Nursing and Mental Health Services* (January 1975).
42. Barry Bricklin and Patricia M. Bricklin. "Psychotherapy, natural: freeing yourself and others from habits that blockade happiness." In Bricklin, *Natural Healing*, pp. 429–449.
43. LeCron, *Self Hypnotism*, pp. 165–166, 198–199.
44. John Feltman. "Raise your serum fun level," *Prevention* (July 1977), pp. 148–155.
45. "How people cope with pain," *Behavior Today* (June 21, 1976), p. 6.
46. LeCron, *Self Hypnotism*, pp. 126–128.
47. "Right in the neck," *Prevention* (December 1978), pp. 89–92.
48. Doris A. Geitgey. "Low back pain." In *ANA Clinical Sessions.* New York: Appleton-Century-Crofts, 1975, pp. 267–278.
49. Merna Dee Galassi and John P. Galassi. *Assert Yourself! How To Be Your Own Person.* New York: Human Sciences Press, 1977, p. 4.
50. Carolyn Chambers Clark. *Assertive Skills For Nurses.* Wakefield, Mass.: Nursing Resources, 1978.
51. Thomas H. Holmes. *Schedule of Recent Experience.* Seattle, Wash.: Department of Psychiatry and Behavioral Sciences, University of Washington School of Medicine, 1976.
52. Irwin Sarason, James H. Johnson, and Judith M. Siegel. "Assessing the impact of life changes: development of the life experiences survey," *Journal of Consulting and Clinical Psychology* 46, no. 5 (1978), pp. 932–946.
53. Barbara Snell Dohrenwend, Larry Krashoff, Alexander R. Askenasy, and Bruce P. Dohrenevend. "Exemplification of a method for scaling life events: The peri life events scale," *Journal of Health and Social Behavior* 19 (June 1978), pp. 205–209.

54. James C. Coleman. "Life stress and maladaptive behavior," *Nursing Digest* (December 1973), pp. 4-15.
55. Jerome K. Meyers, Max Pepper, Jacob L. Lindenthal, and David R. Ostrander. "Life events and mental status," *Nursing Digest* (November 1973), pp. 5-10.
56. Elisabeth Kubler-Ross. *On Death and Dying.* New York: Macmillan, 1969.
57. Richard Schulz and David Aderman. "Clinical research and the stages of dying," *Nursing Digest* (January/February 1976), pp. 47-48.
58. Seymour Shubin. "Cancer widows," *Nursing '78* (April 1978), pp. 56-60.
59. Edith Louise Kowalsky. "Grief: a lost life-style," *American Journal of Nursing* 78, no. 3 (1978), pp. 418-420.
60. Mary Jo Klepser. "Grief—how long does grief go on?" *American Journal of Nursing* 78, no. 3 (1978), pp. 420-428.
61. "Viewpoint on nutrition," Channel 9, New York, March 17, 1979.
62. Marsh Morrison. *The Healthview Newsletter* no. 16 (1978), p. 4.
63. Bricklin, *Natural Healing*, pp. 300-301.
64. Donald M. Vickery. *Life Plan For Your Health.* Reading, Mass.: Addison-Wesley, 1978, pp. 157-158.

5

Caring for Self and Others

This chapter focuses on caring for self and others; balance in these two aspects of caring leads to wellness. People who spend all their time taking care of others and not looking after themselves are bound to experience an imbalance, and likewise, those who choose to focus only on themselves or who do not know how to care for others. Again, as with other dimensions, it is wise to keep in mind that caring needs to be considered in relation to nutrition, fitness, stress reduction, healing, environment, and self-responsibility. Some topics considered in this chapter are: caring/trusting and empathy, saying no, parenting, working effectively in a group, intimate communication, crisis intervention, support networks, and sense of purpose. Figure 5-1 can be used to help you to become attuned to caring for yourself and for others.

CARING/TRUSTING AND EMPATHY

Empathy is intimately tied to caring/trusting. To care deeply for another person (or oneself) implies that you must take a risk, make a commitment. Caring without empathy indicates a lack of respect for the other. It is important to be aware of what you want from a relationship and how you feel. Once you are aware of your own desires and feelings, you can begin to perceive more accurately the thoughts and feelings of those for whom you care.

Thinking that you know what the other person's problem is and just what to do about it is the opposite of empathy, which involves understanding the current feelings of others. Judging others' current feelings based on past experience or the expectation of how they always act (feel, think) is invalid in a caring/trusting relationship. Empathy with others allows you to "borrow" another person's feelings to understand them while still maintaining a separate identity. You can be empathic with a helpless, crying child without resorting to tears and helplessness. Empathy provides a balance between emotional acceptance and intellectual objectivity or separateness.

Empathy provides an emotional mirror for the reflection of others' feelings. Empathic people learn to use the words and language of those they care about and reflect feelings and ideas back [1] to check whether "this is how the other person feels." Advice is not given unless it has been asked for, and then only once there has been an attempt to solve the problem together; behavior is not labeled—for example, as "childish" or "crazy." Instead, they use the tone of voice or mood conveyed by the person they care for. This reflection should not take on the tone, "Here is what you are saying"; it should, instead, be made in a tentative manner, such as, "It sounds as if you're very angry about this," or "It seems as if you're very discouraged."

At this point it may be difficult to know exactly how to teach oneself or others how to be empathic. Creative visualization is often useful in learning how another person might feel. Figure 5-2 gives specific directions for learning how a parent or client might feel about going to live in a nursing home, but the idea can be used for many other situations, such as how a boss might feel, what it feels like to be a child, how a friend might react, and so on.

There are two other crucial skills to be learned, the first of which is active listening. Although listening seems simple and passive, it is difficult to stop trying to solve other people's problems for them, telling them what we would do under similar circumstances, and pooh-poohing the problem by discounting its importance ("What are you worrying about, I've got worse problems than that"). In most conversations, the person who is not speaking is frequently not listening very carefully to what is being said but instead is getting ready to interrupt, preach, moralize, boast, discount what the other has just said, convince, reassure, or give advice. Many conversations sound like double monologues, where both people want to be listened to, but neither is listening to the other. Person B is silent until Person A pauses for breath, and then Person B launches into his or her own topic or style. Sometimes in superficial conversations ("Hello. How are you?" "Fine. Yourself?" "O.K.") people do talk about the same thing, but these are more like rituals with a known outcome than intimate conversations. In other cases, Person A and Person B have their own agenda and may just be waiting for "speaking time," or Person A may have a particular mission—to convince, reassure, give advice—and will attempt to complete that mission despite the fact that it is not helpful to Person B and without listening to and trying to understand what the other person is saying.

On the other hand, in active listening the listener must have a conscious desire to listen attentively without preconceived notions and, from a sense of caring, try to understand not only from the words but also from emotions and body movements what the other person is trying to communicate.

Active listening is an inherent part of the second skill, reflective communication. Reflective communication is "any talk or gesture or attitude that helps another person clarify what he is really thinking and feeling at a given moment, in the depths of his gut" [2]. To be effective, reflective communication must combine a neutral statement of the words and emotional content just conveyed by the other person. This may seem simple, but it is not always easy to do without sounding like a parrot. This kind of communication acknowledges that people may often ask for advice but seldom take it, or if they do, there is no permanent change or growth unless they have come to alter their own way of thinking. People often fail to solve their daily problems because they are limited in their ability to see all their options; they may think they are locked into one solution and may have difficulty seeing others. If you are skilled in reflective communication, you can provide assistance by encouraging them to take responsibility for making decisions yet providing a way for them to see things in a new way by placing a mirror before them.

Reflective communication provides a sounding board against which others learn to be more independent while experiencing a sense of caring, closeness, and help with clarifying their thoughts and feelings, expand their consciousness and wholeness as people, and work out their own solutions.

Figure 5-3 shows the difference between a person who helps another by using reflective communication and another person who pooh-poohs the problem, attempts to solve the problem for the other, taking the problem right back to where it began. Figure 5-4 is an exercise you can use to increase your skill at active listening and reflective communication.

Bricklin and Bricklin suggest the following tips for using reflective communication:

> Phrase comments as statements, not questions. If you use questions, others will think you are dense or hard of hearing.

> Try to rephrase what is said to you in a way that pinpoints both its emotional and verbal content.

> Continue reflective communication as long as it seems helpful. If the person switches to another theme, be sure to switch too; try to stay with where the other person is [3].

SAYING NO

At first glance, caring and saying no appear to have nothing in common. In fact, it is impossible to really care for oneself and others without the ability to say no, to know the limits within which you can be helpful to others, and at what point their demands become harmful to you or them. For example, children need to know the limits within which they can operate to give them the security of knowing where their parents stand; these limits need to be consistent, but ever-expanding, to assist them to grow and be more independent. By saying no, parents also say to children: "I am human, too. I have needs and limits."

At times, spouses, friends, bosses, or others may be very convincing and even threatening if others do not comply with their wishes. Saying no under these conditions requires courage and skill. Some steps to take to increase this skill are:

1. Decide under what conditions it is important to you to say no. Ask what rights do you have as a person. What responsibilities do you have to the other person? To yourself?
2. Dispel counterproductive beliefs about saying no.
3. Use creative visualization to view yourself saying no and feeling good about doing so.
4. When asked to meet a request you have decided not to meet, resist the impulse to blurt out a response. Be aware that you have the right to postpone making a decision for a reasonable length of time.

5. Be sure to sound firm and decisive; others will continue to demand if you sound unsure about your decision.
6. If the other person persists, be persistent in saying no. Remind yourself that you have the right to say no.
7. Resist becoming involved in side arguments. Stick to the issue at hand.

An exercise for practicing saying no is given in Figure 5-5.

PARENTING

Parenting is considered in its larger framework here as any situation where nurturance is given. In fact, you can parent or be nurturing to children, yourself, your spouse or friends, or your own parents. Figures 5-6, 5-7, 5-8, 5-9 [4], and 5-10 [5] provide ways of assessing your values about parenting, making a (more-or-less) rational decision about whether to have a child or not, preparing for parenthood, identifying problems in parenting, and providing your own nurturing/parenting experiences.

Parents who are considering having a baby or adopting a child can often benefit from education classes. No one method seems to offer total benefits. A more useful approach may be one that combines communication skills that enhance parent-child relationships with behavior modifications skills that offer effective control techniques and offer help with specific behavioral problems. These two components will be discussed briefly.

Communication Skills Approach

The communication skills approach is perhaps best exemplified by Dr. Thomas Gordon's, *Parent Effectiveness Training* [6]. Gordon contends there are 12 categories of parental response that lead to low self-esteem in children, low competence/responsibility, and feelings or thoughts about not being understood or accepted. The *nonhelpful* categories are: ordering, directing, and commanding; warning, admonishing, threatening; exhorting, moralizing, preaching; advising, giving solutions or suggestions; lecturing, teaching, giving logical arguments; judging, criticizing, disagreeing, blaming; praising, agreeing; name-calling, ridiculing, shaming, interpreting, analyzing, diagnosing; reassuring, sympathizing, consoling, supporting; probing, questioning, interrogating; withdrawing, distracting, humoring, diverting.

Instead of using comments from these categories, Gordon suggests that parents begin to use "door-openers" or invitations to talk. Figure 5–11 shows some "door-openers." Other kinds of comments Gordon suggests using are "I" messages; these contain "a statement of the parent's feelings about how the child's feelings or behavior affect the parent" [7]. Figure 5–12 compares "I" messages with "You-blaming" messages; the latter close off communication, whereas the former let the child know how his or her parent feels, and put the responsibility for the feeling with the parent.

Gordon agrees that there *will* be parent–child conflicts. For these situations, a no-lose method is suggested. This method is a problem-solving approach that includes the following six steps [8]:

identifying and defining the conflict

stating alternative solutions

evaluating each alternative

choosing a solution

deciding how to implement the solution

evaluating the results

Figure 5–13 gives an illustration of how a parent can use the no-lose method. The communication skills approach is thought to have a preventive as well as a day-to-day effect. For example, adolescents who feel good about themselves, their relationships with their parents (and other significant people in their lives), who can talk about their feelings and consider alternate ways of handling situations are less likely to try to reduce their tension or escape from it through drugs, drinking, and so on [9, 10].

Social Learning Skills Approach

Parents who face problems of fighting, crying, temper tantrums, or refusal to do school work may think the communication skills approach is like "going to war with a squirt gun" [11]. Another approach to parenting is the behavior modification or social learning theory approach.

Controlling the behavior of one's children is part of the socialization process. The social learning skills approach is an attempt to deal with observable, countable behaviors and has proved most successful with specific behavior problems. Parents learn to look at their children's behavior in a systematic way, analyze what is maintaining the behavior in the environment, and plan a strategy to reinforce desirable behavior. Some people question the ethics of controlling children in this way, but there *is* a power imbalance inherent in the parent–child relationship. Behavior is controlled primarily through positives such as praise, hugging, special activities, or concrete rewards such as money or food. Children can increase their self-esteem and learn responsibility through this approach. Democracy can be built into a social learning program by involving the child in setting up the program and negotiating for rewards [12].

The first step in teaching parents (or children) how to use this approach is to help them determine what are *countable* behaviors. Figure 5-14 gives examples of countable and uncountable behaviors. Notice how the column on the left, "Countable Behaviors" can be observed easily, whereas those in the right-hand column cannot be. A simple way to know whether countable behaviors are being listed is to ask, "How will I know if my child has done what I want?"

After the parenting problem is specified in countable behaviors, parents can begin to count the specified behaviors; this period of time, often a week or so, is called the baseline period. During this time, parents merely observe and count the target behaviors, but make no attempt to respond differently to them. This baseline information can later be compared with results obtained for attempting to modify the behaviors. Baseline data can be charted on a graph, or counted in terms of how often the behavior occurs, how long it continues, or how the behavior changes over time. The method used depends on the behavior. Frequency (or how often the behavior occurs) may be most useful for behaviors such as setting the table. Duration (or how long the behavior continues) may be the best measure for behavior such as watching television quietly. Rate (or how the behavior changes over time) is probably most suitable in measuring such things as weight loss.

The next step in decreasing undesirable behavior is to choose rewards and punishments. There are some rewards that can be used with nearly every child—attention, smiles, praise, hugs, television, movies. Rewards cannot be chosen unless the parent establishes control over whether it is dispensed. For example, if the parents let their child watch television whether or not homework has been completed, television is not a good reward.

A principle of social learning that must be observed is that the reward must immediately follow the desired behavior. For example, a reward must be given *every time, right after* the child exhibits the behavior. In some instances, there may be an intermediate step. Tokens, stars, marks on wall charts, and so on, are sometimes used as immediate rewards; the parent and child agree beforehand exactly how many tokens, stars, or marks are needed to be exchanged for one movie, late night out, or whatever. A written contract is often helpful, and Figure 5-15 shows a sample parent–child contract.

Parents can also learn to use verbal and nonverbal positive rewards. They can begin to study, keep close at hand, and learn to use some of the suggestions that appear in Figure 5-16 [13]. There are other rules and principles that need to be followed if a social learning approach is to be successful. Some of these are:

1. State rules positively ("When you finish your homework, you can play outside"; "You can come and eat as soon as you clean your room"; "If you drink your milk, you can have dessert").
2. Plan rewards *prior* to the occurrence and deliver them consistently right after the desired behavior occurs.
3. Specify commands or house rules in the form of statements ("Please go to bed now") rather than as questions ("Will you please go to bed now?").
4. When the child does not comply within the stated period of time, remind the child of the planned reward ("Finish your milk and you'll get dessert") or punishment ("Stop crying or go to your room").
5. Use "time-outs" for the child's inappropriate behavior (choose an area in the house where the child cannot engage in privileges such as eating, talking, playing, or watching television). Set a specific time (usually 3 to 5 minutes) for "time-outs." With children aged 3 to 6, restart the time period if they speak or leave their chair before the time is up. Bernal [14] suggests giving children *one* hard spank and returning them to their chair.
6. Avoid hugging, picking up, physically loving, or nagging the child when he or she misbehaves or immediately after disciplining the child.
7. Give abundant praise during the day, especially when the child is behaving as desired.
8. Spend time teaching the child and having the child practice new ways of behaving; you can demonstrate the appropriate behavior and help the child rehearse; be sure to praise any behavior that

approximates what is desired and to ignore other behaviors. For example, say "That's good, you drank half your glass of milk" *not* "You aren't drinking enough milk."

9.   As the child learns the desired behavior, *gradually* increase the number of points required to obtain a reward. This "fading" procedure can also be used with words; as the child learns the behavior, it can be maintained by only occasional verbal reinforcement.

When two parents are involved with parenting a child, it is wise to have *both* involved in working with a child using a contract and progress sheet. Otherwise, one parent may disagree with the contract and refuse to go along with it. Since social learning depends on consistent rewards, such an approach will be unsuccessful unless all involved are engaged in the program.

Other members of the family can often help parents to be better at parenting. For example, in one family two teenage daughters learned to record independently the frequency of their father's shouting and the amount of time their mother spent with them. Over a period of eight weeks, the daughters rewarded desirable behaviors of their parents [15]. Some ways in which parents can soothe infants and provide them (and themselves) with important sensory learning experiences are the following:

1.   Buy, borrow, or make a cradle and rock the infant regularly.
2.   Invest in a rocker—use it to soothe and stimulate your infant and enhance parents' digestion, circulation, and muscle tone.
3.   Sew or purchase a cloth front-carrying pouch for the small infant, and a hip sling or back-carrying pack for the older infant.
4.   Experiment and find out how much normal activity parents can engage in while carrying the infant.
5.   Avoid use of "L"-shaped infant seats that do not allow the infant's spine to conform to warm, rounded body contours.
6.   Do not be afraid to pick up the baby whenever he or she cries; studies show that those whose cries are consistently responded to as infants are more autonomous at age two and three than those who are left to cry "to teach them independence."
7.   If a child has learning or behavior problems and was not held or rocked as an infant, look into sensory integration therapy.
8.   Find ways parents can enjoy more gentle touching or rhythmic experiences, such as water beds, swings, skipping rope, a porch swing, or folk dancing [16].

BEING AN EFFECTIVE MEMBER OF A GROUP

Another way of caring is shown through the ability to work well in a group. The family is one kind of group you may be involved in. There are also social, supportive groups, teaching/learning groups, and task or work groups (where the focus is on completing a task or attaining a goal). Cooperation and collaboration are needed for effective group work.

There are some common problems that seem to occur in most groups such as overtalkative group members, unequal talking time among members, scapegoating, silence or "the silent treatment," and changes in group composition. Some of these problems are due to unequal or inadequate provision of task and maintenance functions. Members can begin to pay attention to the workings of the groups they participate in and to ask whether they could help this group by:

getting the group moving

keeping the group moving toward its goal

clarifying other's comments or behavior

suggesting ways of accomplishing the goal

pointing out movement toward accomplishing the goal

restating more clearly others' comments

refocusing the group on the task

giving information

giving support to group members who are unsure or anxious

relieving tension

encouraging direct communication

voicing group feeling

agreeing or accepting

helping the group evaluate itself

Some specific examples can show how these functions can help a group. For example, sometimes family or group members talk a lot because they are trying to convince others of the correctness or worthwhileness of their ideas; in this case, providing the function of agreeing/accepting will reduce the talkativeness. Another source of overtalkativeness is an attempt to be recognized or to reduce threat; in this case, reducing tension and providing acceptance—though not necessarily agreement—would help.

Sometimes more specific measures need to be taken to deal with the group problems mentioned earlier. It is always useful to look at a group problem, such as overtalkativeness, as just that, *a group problem.* So-and-so talks too much because others allow it (do not speak up to get the floor) possibly because they do not have the assertive skills necessary for speaking up. In the first instance, one can assume that one person's overtalkativeness serves a purpose in the group and so it is tolerated; on the other hand, overtalkativeness by one person can be viewed as abdication of responsibility by the group members for what happens in the group. Sometimes calling this to the attention of the group helps; for example, "I think we have a problem here with equal talking time; what suggestions do you have for solving this?" In the second instance, where the group shows a lack of assertiveness, members can learn assertive skills in the group or on their own in workshop or counseling experiences.

Scapegoating, another common group problem that may require special approaches, occurs when one or more members of the group are singled out to be targets for hostility or advice. On some level, sometimes an unconscious one, those who are scapegoated agree to accept this role. Sometimes it is the person who fears being rejected or retaliated against and who never says no to others who ends up doing all the work or being blamed for whatever went wrong. In family groups, one of the children may be labeled as the naughty one and be blamed for whatever goes wrong; there may often be conflicts between parents that are not dealt with directly but instead are covered up and disguised as parent–child issues. For example, if a husband is angry with his wife, he may fear confronting her directly; he may siphon off some anger by shouting at his son for not doing his homework. Children are often targets because they are helpless and dependent on their parents and have little recourse other than to accept the role of scapegoat. Parents can learn to listen to their own scapegoating messages and begin to question: "Why am I always picking on one child?" "Why am I reacting so strongly to what that child does?" "Would I react so strongly if someone else did the same thing he or she is doing?" "What issues between my wife and me am I ignoring?" "Why can't I express my anger directly to the person I am angry with?" "How can I learn to use my anger more constructively so I feel better and my child doesn't suffer?"

In groups other than family groups, members can also begin to question their blaming messages. If group members have assertive skills, scapegoating is unlikely to occur because each person takes responsibility for his or her own thoughts, feelings, and actions. If group members do not have these skills, they can obtain them.

Sometimes family members use the "silent treatment" with each other as a way of retaliating against or punishing each other. If all members had assertive skills, they would be able to use words to express their anger rather than indirect, nonverbal messages such as silence. These angry silences are not constructive in any group, and voicing group feeling (a maintenance function) is one way of intervening. Other silences, such as thoughtful or sad ones, can be helpful in a group, and individuals need to learn how to tolerate these kinds of silences so the group can benefit from thinking or grieving.

When one member comes into or leaves a group, there is usually a period of adjustment. Some situations in which this may occur are if a grandmother comes to live with the family, if a child dies or is born; if a husband and father remarries, or if an employee gets a new boss. There are many other situations where group composition changes. Whenever there is a change, the group's ability to work effectively changes. New members can be eased into a group by preparing both the new member and the group. It is always wise to discuss the new addition and the possible fears, anticipations, and consequences of entering or having a new person enter the group. Some questions to use in this regard are: "What changes do you anticipate?" "What concerns do you have about entering (having a new person enter) the group (family, unit, job, etc.)?" "What problems do you anticipate?" New members can also benefit from specific information regarding rules, procedures, rituals, or expectations for behavior in the group. In addition to this preparation for the entry of a new person, group members can also try to keep open to signs of reaction to the expected changes from anyone concerned; the more openly the group members can talk about the changes and problem-solve, the more successful the change is likely to be.

When one or more persons leave a group—be it a family or a work group—there are bound to be strong feelings, such as sadness, anger, rejection, longing, relief, and accomplishment. The more intense the relationship of the leaving member to the group, the stronger will be the feelings. The better the group and the leaving member can discuss and feel accepted in having these feelings, the more likely will it be that they will separate without carrying unresolved feelings into future relationships. One comment groups can learn to use when a member will be leaving is: "We have feelings about your leaving and we'd like to talk about them with you."

Many groups may feel unable to discuss their feelings, and they may request or need help from a health practitioner who is skilled in working with group processes.

INTIMATE COMMUNICATION

Communication in work or social groups is often more superficial than intimate. Bach and Goldberg suggest that people who marry or who have ongoing, intense one-to-one relationships confront problems of distance/closeness, centricity, power struggles, trust formation, preservation of self, and social boundaries [17]. Figure 5-17 lists some of the questions couples need to ask if they want to enhance their relationships [18].

People who are involved in intimate relationships will sooner or later become angry with one another. Often, people do not know constructive ways of releasing their anger; when no constructive outlet is available, anger may be released in violence or may go underground and emerge in seemingly unrelated violent outbursts, in controlling or blaming behaviors, or in pressures to feel guilty. Bach and Goldberg also suggest a number of rituals that can be used to release anger in a constructive way. It is suggested that these exercises be used when there is not time to deal with the anger at the time it occurred and when people are afraid of their own anger and require a structured framework within which to practice release of anger.

One ritual is to set aside a specific time each day for structured release of anger. Each family member or partner is given time to vent his or her frustrations, resentments, and angers. Listeners provide an attentive audience but do *not* respond to any feelings that are expressed.

Another ritual helps people to hear angry insults without responding. In this exercise, participants consent not to take the exchange literally and agree that there will be no physical violence. Partners set aside a specified period, usually two to five minutes, stand face to face, and scream insults at one another while not listening to the other or responding to the other's comments.

Another ritual for release of anger also requires mutual consent. The initiator has a grievance and wants to scold the other person; the content of the offense is shared, and the offender agrees to accept the one-way scolding. A time limit of one or two minutes is agreed on. The initiator then proceeds to scold the offender, while the offender sits quietly listening. The offender can then ask for clarification about the offense but cannot counter or defend. If the offender agrees to accept responsibility for the offense, he or she can request a "doghouse release" to reestablish good relations.

Another ritualistic release of feeling is an "attraction–reservation" exercise, where participants each share their reaction to an aspect of the other person they find attractive and one that leads to their withdrawal from contact. An example of how this might be done is, "I like it when you come up to me and hug me, but I feel very distant from you and fed up when you nag me about cleaning the stove."

For relationships between a definitely dominant and a submissive person, Bach and Goldberg suggest a ritualistic role reversal. In this exercise, the dominant one agrees to play the submissive or "slave" role, while putting certain limits to the requests the "master" can make, for example, "I will fan you as you sit in your soft chair, but I will not kiss your foot."

A crucial way of releasing anger constructively and negotiating for change is described by Bach and Goldberg in "The Fair Fight" [19]. The ritual takes place within a group of supportive observers; this coaching period is used to help define the grievance, construct a demand for change using "I" statements, and help the offender to practice resisting the demand using "I" or "we-collaborative" comments. Once the coaching is completed, the observers step back and watch. The initiator then states his or her "beef" and the feelings attached to it. Once the grievance has been expressed, neither initiator nor fight partner can express him- or herself without first reporting back what was just heard. Observers are expected to comment whenever they hear a distorted paraphrase or repeat of what was said; comments to use are, "I think I heard Jim say. . . ." or "I didn't hear Sally quite that way; what I heard was. . . ." Next, the initiator makes a demand for change related to expected action ("I want to see more of you"), not of attitude ("You don't love me"). At this point the partner has a chance to respond to both the grievance and the demand for change by telling his or her side. This is followed by a discussion where each person expresses him- or herself in simple, direct terms, using "I" or "we-collaborative" statements; during this step, each person must repeat what has just been said by the other person before stating a new comment. Then the fight partner either accepts the demand for change, rejects it, or negotiates conditions for a partial change. Agreement is reached and stated in clear, direct terms. Now the observers move into action and rate each partner with pluses for fair fighting behaviors (leveling, fairness, genuine emotion, willingness to take responsibility, humor that produces relief or closeness, undistorted feedback, specific statements, here-and-now statements, willingness to be flexible and open to change, and ability to confront messages that confuse because they contain loving *and* rejecting messages) or minuses for fight behaviors that are not fair (contrived messages or manipulation, attempts to devastate the other, detachment or phony feeling expression, blaming, sarcasm or putdowns, distortion in repeating the other's statements, vague comments, bringing up irrelevant issues or allegations from the past, remaining rigid while expecting the other person to change, giving or overlooking statements that confuse because they contain both rejecting and loving messages).

Another ritual allows for a more physical release of anger. In this exercise, participants hit each other with bataca bats (bats are cloth-covered and filled with soft material). Soft pillows could also be used. No one is hurt, and a great release of aggression can be accomplished [20].

Another area of intimate communication relates to sexual satisfaction. Partners need to ask each other some of the questions that appear in Figure 5-18 if they hope to have a satisfying sexual relationship. Figure 5-19 contains directions for a creative visualization exercise to enhance sexual fulfillment. People who wish more specific exercises for enhancing their sexual relationships can refer to the Appendix, Wellness Resources.

CRISIS INTERVENTION

A crisis is a turning-point, a time when old methods of coping do not seem to work. People who are in crisis often feel helpless and unable to take action on their own to solve their problems. However, many crisis points can be anticipated and, if prepared for, a crisis can be averted. Developmental crises are especially available for preventive action, since they are well-known events. Figure 5-20 presents examples of developmental or life-transitional crises; some may require help from others, while some may be prepared for by the individual [21]. Figure 5-21 gives information about ways people have found useful in coping with problematic life circumstances; perhaps some of these can be used by you as a way of preventing crises [22, 23].

You may also be able to do your own crisis intervention in part by beginning to evaluate the problem. Some questions you can ask yourself to begin sorting out whether additional help is needed are:

What is the problem?

Does this problem have an obvious cause? (See Figure 5–20.)

Have I tried everything I can think of to solve the problem?

Has the problem gone on for a short time, or has it persisted for long?

How severe and unusual does this problem seem to me?

How much distress is this problem causing me? My family? My friends?

Am I reacting to a new or tense situation that could be throwing me into a crisis?

Am I under other stresses that might be leading me to blowing this situation up out of proportion?

Do I have a difficult time asking for help with this situation?

Even though I may have difficulty asking for help, do I really need it now?

What friends or family members can I talk to to help me clarify what kind of help I need?

What information regarding help can I find in the yellow pages of my phone book?

Whom do I know that has (had) a similar problem and whom I can call to give me some tips about how to handle this?

What questions or information do I need to write down so I won't forget problems, solutions, contacts, or people to get in touch with?

How can I be persistent and continue to try to make contact with others when I need help, even if I keep getting recorded phone messages, no answer, or no positive response when I try to make contact?

Is there a hotline number I can call for help, and can the operator or the yellow pages help me find the number?

Whom can I ask to sit with me while I make phone calls, to look up agencies, to sit with my children, or to go with me to an agency?

Even if agencies or individuals cannot help me, can they refer me to someone who can?

If I can't make any headway with an agency representative, can I speak to his or her supervisor as a way of getting help with the matter?

If helpers or things I read seem to discount my experiences as invalid, how can I reassure myself that my feelings and perceptions are justified?

Rather than waiting until problems arise, you can begin to become familiar with resources in your community. In addition, you can keep at hand the telephone numbers of friends and professionals who can be contacted for support or to provide ideas regarding additional resources.

SUPPORT NETWORKS

The family often serves as a support network when one family member needs help. Some people do not have families that are supportive, while others do not have families. In these cases, individuals must learn how to develop their own sources of support.

Neighborhoods and workplaces are often places where support can be developed, where people can talk about themselves, share experiences and ideas, and get support. Those who are parents can also develop support through sharing carpools, babysitting tasks, play groups, and ideas about childcare with other parents. More and more people are realizing that health care systems rarely provide opportunities for people to discover how they share common experiences, how to deal with common problems, how to learn new skills or find where to go to learn these skills, and how to get emotional and practical support from a group so changes can be made. When health care systems do not offer these experiences, you can turn to (or develop) self-help support groups or intentional family groups. Pregnant women or people who have chronic illnesses, devastating surgery, or parenting or other problems can form their own support groups, with or without professional guidance. Intentional families are developed by people who do not have families. They live in separate homes and have their own friends, but if someone needs help with work, childrearing, holidays, or other problems, the "family" rallies around. Sometimes intentional families are structured by religious or health care workers. Others develop on their own.

People need to realize that therapists, doctors, and nurses can offer enormous technical help, but it is another mother who can help with day-to-day issues of parenting, or another person with multiple sclerosis who can help with the day-to-day issues of living. Individuals need to be encouraged and assisted to set up their own support networks.

The importance of support goes far beyond the need for help when trouble arises. James J. Lynch, Professor of Psychology and Scientific Director of the Psychosomatic Clinic at the School of Medicine at the University of Maryland, contends that social isolation, grief, and chronic loneliness predispose people to major illnesses such as heart attacks. What is more, once lonely people, or those who live alone, are hospitalized, they tend to remain in the hospital longer (13.5 days as opposed to 8.5 days for the average married individual) [24].

Friendships, marriages, and intimate relationships all seem to be essential elements of support for people on a day-to-day basis. They can provide help through daily frustrations that pile up, such as getting a parking ticket, being "chewed out" by a boss, losing a credit card, and the myriad frustrating experiences everyone has to adapt to. Significant others can say directly or indirectly, "I understand your frustration, and I accept you when you are frustrated or upset." In this way, other people serve as buffers against daily stress. An ongoing friendship "provides a continuous reflection . . . as beneficial mirrors" [25].

Lawrence J. Weiss, a research psychologist and gerontologist, suggests specific ways of building supports [26]:

Develop a *desire* to meet people.

Find voluntary or paid work that "turns you on"—the chances are the people there will turn you on, too.

Be receptive to other people; reach out to them.

Smile at people, say hello, or make a positive comment about their appearance or behavior.

Develop empathy skills so you can get to know others better and be helpful to them.

Force yourself to be in situations where you will come in contact with others.

DEVELOPING A SENSE OF PURPOSE

It is not unusual to hear of two people both of whom have the same illness and the same chance for recovery: one dies, the other lives. Doctors and nurses often report seeing individuals in the hospital who have a good chance for recovery, but who seem to give up and die. Lawrence LeShan, an experimental psychologist and research specialist, offers evidence to show why some individuals get cancer while others do not, and why some cancer victims are able to fight successfully for their lives while others rapidly succumb to the disease [27]. He found the following characteristics of those who developed cancer [28]:

a marked amount of self-dislike and lack of respect for their accomplishments

a block in their ability to express hostility in their own defense

inability to express or be aware of what they really wanted out of life

a hopelessness about ever achieving any meaning, zest, or validity as a person

a sense of aloneness and despair that excludes the possibility of satisfying relationships with others

a feeling of doing and being nothing

a feeling that relationships will ultimately bring pain and dissapointment

a sense that time or action cannot change things since to be oneself is to be rejected

a feeling that death will provide escape from despair

thoughts that cancer is a confirmation the sick person was hopeless and the solution for their problem is getting rid of themselves

LeShan [29] suggests that people who have cancer—and perhaps those susceptible to developing cancer—must have their positive drives freed by relating to someone who views them as positive and capable of developing. Healing occurs when people express themselves in ways that are natural to them. The less they are themselves, the greater stress is placed on them and the greater is the tendency toward illness. Figure 5-22 presents some questions you can use to examine your life purpose, to care for yourself, and possibly to ward off illness [30].

Figure 5–1   Caring/Trusting*

	Always	Some-times	Never	I'm trying	This is new to me, but something I'd like to consider
1. Do I try to be who I am, not who others want me to be?					
2. Am I always trying to discover what I want and feel?					
3. Do I value the unique and special things about me?					
4. Do I try to allow others to be who they are—*not* who I want them to be?					
5. Do I take full responsibility for my thoughts, feelings, and actions?					
6. Do I show my inner feelings to others without masking the message?					
7. Do I clearly convey my motives to others, rather than sugar-coating them or denying that I have any?					
8. Even in my work role, do I try to respond as a unique person in each situation?					

Figure 5–1 /// 223

	Always	Some-times	Never	I'm trying	This is new to me, but something I'd like to consider
9. Do I abstain from categorizing myself to others?					
10. When I am with people, do I focus on my immediate relation-ship with them—not on meaningless chitchat?					
11. When I feel myself becoming defensive with others, do I try to discover how I can join them and collaborate with them?					
12. Do I try to enter each situation with an openness and lack of expectation, not with anticipations, or strategies of influence or manipulation?					
13. Do I show my feelings to others?					
14. Do I cite specific instances, events, or people (rather than ramble on in a generalized, depersonal-ized way)?					
15. When I am with people, do I try to experience the feelings I am having, rather than analying them, talking about					

(continued)

Figure 5–1   (continued)

	Always	Some-times	Never	I'm trying	This is new to me, but something I'd like to consider
them, telling stories or jokes, asking a lot of questions, or escaping into humor?					
16. Am I totally involved with what is happening between me and others at the moment, rather than thinking about what is going to happen or what has happened earlier?					
17. Do I let others see my vulnerability, hidden strengths, biases, and preferences?					
18. Do I let others know that I, too, am fearful about trusting?					
19. Do I touch others and allow them to touch me physically, emotionally, and spiritually?					
20. Do I let others know I value them by sharing my most precious gift, my undivided attention, with them?					
21. Do I trust my own intuition, body wants, rhythms?					
22. Do I care for and nurture my mind/body?					

Figure 5-1 /// 225

	Always	Some-times	Never	I'm trying	This is new to me, but something I'd like to consider
23. Do I focus my energy on being what I want to be?					
24. Do I discover what is blocking me from wellness and focus my energy on removing the barriers?					
25. Do I try to create the world inside and around me?					
26. Do I work with others to coauthor our experience?					
27. Do I allow me to be me and others to be themselves without overmanaging or over-controlling what happens?					
28. Do I focus my energy on what is essential to my wellness?					
29. Am I part of a community and/or family group whose members care about each other?					
30. Do I perceive myself to be a total, whole person, yet interdependent with all others?					
31. Do I try to create a climate of trust and openness with others?					

*Based on ideas presented by Jack Gibb in *Trust: A New View of Personal and Organizational Development.* Los Angeles: Guild of Tutors Press, 1978.

Figure 5–2   Creative Visualization: Becoming the Other Person

---

Step 1:   Allow yourself to relax fully. Use one of the relaxation exercises in Chapter 3.

Step 2:   Take yourself to a deep inner place where you are centered and open to information from yourself.

Step 3:   Choose an age between 65 and 85. See yourself as more or less healthy and as an adult. Gradually see yourself starting to be treated by others as if you were a child, unable to make decisions. Look at your body and notice its aches and pains, its wrinkles, its slowed-down pace. You know you forget things occasionally and tend to live in the past, but your family begins to look at you with puzzled looks, frowns, and frustration. One day they tell you they are taking you for a drive, and you end up at a nursing home. You try to leave when they do, but the nurse gives you a sedative and puts you to bed. You can't sleep because other residents come into your room and ask you how they can get home or shout at their family members loudly from their own rooms. You have a roommate who is blind but gets up constantly during the night to stumble past your bed toward the bathroom. The food is very starchy and salty, and the doctor has taken you off the multivitamin you used to take. It is always very warm and stuffy in the nursing home, and you feel constantly tired and fatigued. You are able to get close to some residents, but they die or go home. Your family comes to see you less and less often, and when they do there is constant tension because you are angry with them, and they act guilty and frustrated with you. Allow yourself to feel the isolation and other anti-wellness effects of the nursing home.

Step 4:   Slowly bring yourself back to the here-and-now, realizing that you were only imagining yourself to be a resident of the nursing home.

Step 5:   Ask yourself the following questions:

1.   What was your experience like?

2.   What did you learn about how it might feel to be a resident in a nursing home?

3.   What could you do to enhance the wellness of residents in such a setting?

Figure 5–3 /// 227

Figure 5–3   Learning to Notice Your Listening and Reflective Skills

---

Step 1:   Choose a three- to five-minute dialogue you are about to have.

Step 2:   Tape record it (with permission), or ask a neutral person to record *your* comments, tone of voice, and gestures.

Step 3:   Analyze your listening skill by asking the following questions:

    A.   What was I doing while the other person was speaking?

    B.   Which of the following did my remarks convey?

        1.   an interruption of the other's statement

        2.   a "preach" or a "speech"

        3.   moral slogans

        4.   bragging about my accomplishments or negative experiences

        5.   a discounting of what the other said

        6.   an attempt to convince the other person

        7.   an attempt to cheer up or reassure

        8.   advice about what the other person should do

        9.   none of these; I was listening and reflecting back what was said

    C.   Why couldn't I just listen to the other person?

Step 4:   (optional) If you had difficulty seeing what your remarks convey, ask your recorder or a skilled listener what your comments sound like to him or her. Get into a good discussion and description of *exactly* what he or she noticed about your listening skills, and try to focus on *listening.*

Step 5:   Repeat Steps 1 through 3 until you consistently answer No. 9 to Step 3B.

Step 6:   (optional) If possible, videotape several short interchanges with another person, and ask him or her to give you some feedback on exactly what you conveyed. Use the questions under Step 3B to obtain feedback.

(continued)

Figure 5-3 (continued)

Step 7: Keep a record of situations where you did not listen. Write down at least three situations. Reconstruct each situation and compare them according to the following components: What was being discussed; what the other person was doing; what you were doing, thinking, and feeling; how you responded; what happened between the two of you when you stopped listening.*

Step 8: Choose three situations where you will have time to spend time listening to another person. Try to listen attentively by: looking at the person with interest (not staring), hearing his or her comments through before giving advice; making comments that encourage the other to go on, such as, "uh-huh," "go on," or "tell me more about that"; asking questions that help the other person to problem-solve, such as, "What do *you* think about that?" or "What have you tried to solve that?" Make mental notes for yourself about how the other person may feel, how his or her voice sounds, and any gestures or postures made that may be related to what is being said.

*This step was developed in collaboration with Susan DiFabio, RN, MS.

Reflective communication

person A: "I don't know what I'm going to do! My daughter, Sarah, just will not go out and get a job!" (sounding annoyed and frustrated)

person B: "It's really very annoying when your daughter doesn't get a job."

person A: "Yes, I've tried everything I can think of; got any ideas?"

person B: "You have tried *everything* you can think of?"

person A: "Well, I've tried not giving her her allowance, and hollering at her. Those didn't work, so I went back to giving her an allowance." (At this point the client is moving past the impasse.)

person B: "So you tried two things, and neither one worked. But you changed your mind about not giving Sarah her allowance."

person A: "Do you think Sarah is confused by that? Maybe I shouldn't have reversed. Or maybe I could stick with the no allowance a little longer."

person B: "So you think there is a possibility that Sarah may be confused by the reversal, and that you do have some options to try."

Nonempathic communication

person A: "I don't know what I'm going to do! My daughter just will not go out and get a job!" (sounding annoyed and frustrated)

person B: "You think you've got it bad! My son is on dope."

person A: "Kids are really something. If Sarah would only try."

person B: "I think you should tell her to get a job or move out."

person A: "But I'd feel so guilty."

person B: "If I were you, I wouldn't feel guilty. After all, look at how much you've done for her."

person A: "Yes, but I can't just throw her out on the street. Oh, what am I going to do?!"

Figure 5-5 Practice in Saying No

Step 1:   Experiment with saying no until you feel comfortable saying it.

Step 2:   Ask a friend or family member to listen to your no and tell you whether you sound convincing. Ask that person for tips on how you could sound firmer.

Step 3:   Choose one or more of the statements below, and practice saying it until you sound decisive:

1. No, I cannot help you with that now.

2. No, you cannot borrow my car (notes, clothes, money).

3. No, I cannot work overtime today.

4. No, I can't decide that now. I'll think it over and let you know my decision on Monday morning.

5. No, I won't change my mind.

Step 4:   List one or two situations in which you wish to say no. Practice saying no. It may be useful to tape your statements and then to play them back to see how decisive you sound.

Figure 5-6 /// 231

Figure 5-6   Clarifying Values about Parenting

Directions:

Read the statements below, and check where you are in your values about parenting.

		Yes	No	Some-times
1.	I know how parenting fits in with my overall life—my work, relationships, social and political concerns, my own childhood experiences, and my sense of my own self	......	......	....
2.	I have tried to examine how society shapes my experiences as a parent	......	......	....
3.	I know when I need nurturance or parenting myself *and* where to go to get it	......	......	....
4.	I realize that being a parent or a source of nurturance for others can lead to my feeling conflicted, entrapped, uncertain, more stimulated, and more whole as a person	......	......	....
5.	I can accept the fact that I can never be the mythical perfect parent	......	......	....
6.	I realize it is creative for all concerned that while I am parenting I am also making sure I get my own needs met as a full human being who is only partly parent	......	......	....
7.	I try not to make those whom I parent extensions of myself; we each have our own identity to assert and accept	......	......	....
8.	I know that those whom I parent will never be neglected if I meet my own needs for support, friendship, work, security, health care, play, and time alone	......	......	....
9.	As a parent, I realize I have specific responsibilities for the other person and, therefore, a right to set limits on his or her behavior	......	......	....

(continued)

Figure 5-6 (continued)

	Yes	No	Some-times
10. (For female parents) I feel comfortable negotiating family arrangements so I don't end up doing all the housework, struggling to get time for myself, or exploring other facets of me	......	......	....
11. (For male parents) I allow my child-oriented, nurturing side to come out	......	......	....
12. I can negotiate with my workplace to be respected as a parent by achieving flexible work hours, day care, maternity or paternity leaves, and so on	......	......	....
13. I have considered the idea that parenting may often be less a pleasure and more something to be endured and resented and an experience that may lead to feeling frustrated	......	......	....
14. I realize that much as I may want a child, during pregnancy or after delivery I may regret having chosen to have a child; I also realize that this is normal and an O.K. reaction	......	......	....

Figure 5–7 /// 233

Figure 5–7   Deciding to Have a Child

Directions:

Read the questions below, ponder them, and use them in your decision-making process. Prospective parents can do this exercise separately and then discuss the results together. Decide which of your answers, pressures, or experiences should influence you, which you should ignore, and for which you need help from a professional.

1. What positive and negative childhood memories influence my decision about having a child?
2. What movies, books, television shows, or friends' comments or experiences influence my decision about having a child?
3. What do I think I would miss if I decided not to have a child?
4. What are the advantages of having a child?
5. What pressures from family or friends are influencing my decision to have a child?
6. Do I have the energy and sense of responsibility necessary for caring for a child?
7. How will having children affect my career?
8. How willing am I to share in caring for a child?
9. How willing am I to have a child and be the primary care giver if my partner does not really care to have a child?
10. Am I choosing to have a child simply as a defiant act or as a way to get away from my parents or prove something?
11. Have I thought about how difficult it will be for me and my partner to spend time together when the child is small?
12. Am I willing to give up special time or nurturance from my partner in order to use our energy to care for a child?
13. Am I willing to put up with a new set of restrictions on my mobility and freedom in exchange for a child?
14. Am I willing to plan a supportive network of friends, family, babysitters, health care workers, and playmates for the child?
15. Do I know what hereditary diseases (or other problems) I will be encountering as a result of choosing to have a child now?
16. Have I thought about how my experiences as a child may influence my ability to be a parent? What fears or confidence do I have in myself because of my experiences while growing up? For example, how was I punished as a child?

Figure 5–8 Looking Forward to Parenthood

Directions:

This exercise can be used with women and their partners who are sharing a birthing experience. These statements can be thought about individually and then shared in a caring, active listening way. Omit statements that do not seem to apply to you.

1. I often wonder what I will be like as a parent; at these times, the following thoughts and feelings come to mind:

2. When I think about being a parent, I worry about the following things:

3. I wonder how children will change my life; some thoughts I have on the subject are:

4. I think that parenthood will ask a lot of me, let me express new feelings and develop new skills; some thoughts I have about this are:

5. Parenthood will put me in a new relationship with my parents; I think this will have the following effect(s):

6. I've been thinking about the physical changes pregnancy brings (morning sickness, loss of balance, fatigue, frequent urination, protruding stomach, stretch marks, varicose veins), and I have the following reactions:

7. I've thought about how I want the birth to occur, and this is how I picture it:

8. I worry about developing a bond with my child, even though I *know* it takes time to do so; I plan to do the following things to develop this bond:

Figure 5–8 /// 235

9. I know I (my partner) may lose my (her) strength, my (her) clothes size, my (her) sexual self-image, and maybe my (her) job and economic independence; all of these changes can lead to postpartum "blues." To cope with this, we plan to get good information on exercise, diet, finding household and child-care help, and sharing with my partner. My reactions to this problem are:

10. I know I may be moody or irritable after the baby comes. I want to take the following measures to cope with these feelings so I don't take them out on my partner or others:

11. I know I may need parenting or nurturing myself when I will be giving so much to the baby; thoughts I have on this subject are:

12. I worry somewhat about scary situations like convulsions, diarrhea, or that the baby might cry on and on when there seems no reason for it; some reactions and ideas for solving this problem are:

13. I think about playing with the baby and I picture myself:

14. I think about how I can share the baby with my parents; some ideas I have are:

15. When I think about leaving the baby, I feel somewhat guilty or selfish at times; things I want to share with my partner (or a trusted friend) about this are:

Figure 5–9 Problems in Parenting

Directions:

Check the problems you have or anticipate having as a parent. Discuss the problems with a health care worker whom you trust, or begin a self-help group for parents.

		Yes	No

Infancy

1. When I look at my child, it looks ugly and repulsive ....

2. My child's odor, vomitus, bowel movements, drooling, or sucking are revolting to me ....

3. I find myself being preoccupied or annoyed with the odor, type, or number of bowel movements my child has ....

4. I worry that I'm not holding my child right; I feel so awkward, and don't know how to approach the baby ....

5. I worry that my baby moves too much (or too little) or is too tense (or sleepy) ....

6. I feel uncomfortable talking or cooing to my baby ....

7. Sometimes I worry that my baby might be defective, ill, or unable to love ....

8. I seem to need constant reassurance that my baby is normal ....

9. I never seem to know whether my baby is hungry, tired, needs to be held, or what is wrong ....

10. I seem to rush right in when the baby starts to cry and "do something" ....

11. I let the baby cry and cry most of the time, even though it drives me crazy and I feel like screaming sometimes, but I don't want to spoil the child ....

12. Sometimes I expect my baby to comfort me ....

13. I can't seem to develop outside interests or people I can count on for support ....

Figure 5-9 /// 237

	Yes	No

14. Sometimes I find my fear and irritation escalating when I think about or look at my demanding child   ....

15. Sometimes I feel pulled between my sexual needs and the baby's needs   ....

Childhood

16. I seem to have no way to vent my angry feelings toward my child   ....

17. I want to help my child become more independent, but it takes so much longer to let them do it themselves   ....

18. My child seems to want independence, but when I let him (her) try, he (she) gets so frustrated and wants help; I feel like a human Yo-Yo   ....

19. My child seems to resent my relationships with others and always tries to interfere; sometimes I get so angry I don't know what to do   ....

20. I find it hard to set limits with my child. I wonder whether scolding, ordering, and bossing is all there is to being a parent   ....

21. Sometimes I feel guilty or selfish when I tell my child "no"   ....

22. My child can get me to give in if he (she) calls me "stupid," throws a temper tantrum, or tells me I'm bad   ....

23. I feel guilty when I leave my child to go to work or to get away for a while for some time to myself or for some adult social activity   ....

24. Sometimes the way my parents held me back or pushed me ahead interferes with my ability to judge how independent I can allow my child to be   ....

25. I find it hard to tolerate my children's defeats, hurts, or mistakes; I guess I want to protect them too much   ....

(continued)

Figure 5–9 **(continued)**

	Yes	No
26. When my child says "so-and-so's mother lets *her* do it!" I feel angry, hurt, and/or unsure about my ability to be a parent	......	......
27. I find it difficult to teach my child rules for caring for themselves and at the same time let it be known that I don't have all the answers	......	......
28. I have a hard time teaching my child to respect others and themselves, and how to act responsibly	......	......
29. I find that my ideas about how to raise my child clash with my partner's	......	......
30. Sometimes I find it difficult to be open and honest about my thoughts and feelings with my child	......	......
31. I find it difficult to explain to my child that I need the companionship and love of adults	......	......
32. Sometimes I find it difficult to be affectionate with my partner when my child is around, even though I would like to be	......	......
33. My child is beginning to desire privacy and separateness, and this leads to my discomfort; I'm not sure how to deal with it	......	......

Teenage Years

34. Sometimes my teenager challenges my ideas and behaves in ways I find intolerable	......	......
35. My teenager seems to be exploring too many things too quickly	......	......
36. I worry that my teenager may be experimenting with sex, drugs, alcohol, or other unsafe situations	......	......
37. My teenager has suddenly become very silent and stopped sharing things with me; I worry about this	......	......

Figure 5–9 /// 239

		Yes	No
38.	I try to stay in touch with what is going on with my teenager while still giving him (her) privacy; I think I'm failing at this	......	......
39.	I find myself competing with my teenager for his or her friends	......	......
40.	I find myself feeling sad and empty when I think my teenager will soon be leaving home; sometimes I become even more protective when I feel this way	......	......
41.	I find it difficult to agree with my partner about how to raise my teenager	......	......
42.	I have trouble talking to or being with my partner without my teenager interrupting or interfering	......	......
43.	I often feel uncertain about how to offer help to my teenager	......	......
44.	I find it difficult to keep to limits I have set for my teenager; sometimes I set very strict rules and other times I overlook it when my teenager breaks a rule	......	......
45.	I find it difficult not to get caught up in my teenager's day-to-day ups and downs	......	......
46.	I have difficulty maintaining my self-esteem when my teenager puts me down	......	......

Figure 5-10   Providing Your Own Parenting [5]

Step 1:   Relax your body using a relaxation exercise.

Step 2:   Close your eyes and imagine yourself in a comforting, quiet place. Go wherever you feel good.

Step 3:   Imagine that your nurturing parent is coming to visit you. Imagine what he or she looks like. Visit this person and listen to the loving, caring, and nurturing things this person has to say.

Step 4:   Write down some of the caring and nurturing comments your nurturing parent said to you. If you have trouble getting in touch with these messages, you might choose to draw the effects of a nurturing message or to draw how you would be (physically) in relation to your nurturing parent's message.

Step 5:   Picture yourself as a child. Write, draw, say aloud, or act out how a parent could be nurturing to you. Use child-like expressions to convey the messages, such as "Holds me gently," "Hugs me warmly," "Loves me," "Understands my hurt," "I love you as you are," "You are beautiful to me." (Be sure to use positive messages; exclude negative ones such as, "You are not ugly.")

Step 6:   (optional) Find a partner, and share your list, drawing, or pantomine. Say the words, share the drawing, or act the nurturance in a loving, tender way. Allow yourself to listen fully to your own and your partner's needs for parenting. If you like, ask your partner to say or do the things you consider nurturing; allow yourself to bask in good feelings about being parented. Be sure you choose a partner who *wants* to be nurturing, not one who feels obligated to do so.

Step 7:   Refer to your list or drawing often. Provide your own parenting by nurturing yourself.

Figure 5–11 /// 241

Figure 5–11   Some "Door-Openers"

Umm-hm

I see.

Go on.

Tell my exactly what happened.

I'm listening.

I'd like to hear more.

Let's talk about this.

Let's try to work this out.

Sounds important.

Let's discuss it more.

Let's see if we can figure this out together.

I want to hear your views.

I'd like to listen.

I'm interested in hearing what you have to say.

Tell me more.

And then what happened?

Start at the beginning and tell me the whole story.

Figure 5-12 "I" and "You-Blaming" Messages

"I" messages	*"You-blaming" messages*
I am upset that your chores aren't finished.	I am upset that you have been *neglectful* of your chores.
(Parent owns the feeling of upset; makes neutral statement about chores not being completed.)	(Underlying message: You are neglectful; this is a you-blaming message masquerading as an "I" message.)
Billy, I get scared when you hit your brother. I'm afraid he will be badly hurt.	Don't you dare hit your brother again; I'll hit you and see how you like it!
(Parent owns the feeling of fright; lets Billy know he could hurt his brother badly.)	(Parent threatens Billy and conceals her own fear by threatening to attack herself.)
I don't like being kicked; it hurts me.	You bad girl; don't you ever kick me again!
(Parent states feeling and lets child know being kicked hurts.)	(Parent blames daughter and labels her as a bad girl.)
I'm in a hurry, and I don't have time to play.	You're a naughty boy!
(Parent "clues" son in to the situation.)	(Parent labels son as naughty but does not clarify why she does not want to play now.)
I feel let down; I thought we had agreed you would clean your room.	You should be ashamed of yourself! This room is a pigsty!
(Parent owns the feeling of being let down and restates their verbal agreement, leaving the responsibility for action with the child.)	(Parent discounts own feeling and blames child; no suggestion for how the issue is to be dealt with is given.)

Figure 5-13 /// 243

Figure 5-13   Using the No-Lose Method

Parent:	I feel it is unfair for me to do all the housework. I'd like some help from you.
Child:	Silence.
Parent:	I am really serious about finding a solution to this that both of us can accept.
Child:	Well I'm not helping (starts crying and runs to his room).
Parent:	(goes after child) I'm darned angry at you now. I want to work this out and you run away. I feel I'm being treated unfairly. I don't want you to lose on this, but I don't want to lose either. Come back to the table so we can work out a solution where we will both win.
Child:	(dries tears, returns to table)
Parent:	What suggestions do you have for the housework problem?
Child:	Why don't you hire someone else to do it.
Parent:	O.K., that's a possibility. First we'll write down all solutions. I'll add "rotate chores" as another possibility.
Child:	I could help with the dishes, but I won't take out the garbage.
Parent:	O.K., that's another solution—divide chores by who wants to do what. I can't think of any more solutions, can you?
Child:	No.
Parent:	O.K. Let's see how each one might work. If we hire someone, that means fewer movies and snacks for the family. I just can't afford to pay for both.
Child:	I like the movies and snacks. I don't want to give those up. What's the next solution? Rotate chores? Well, some chores I just don't like, so that's not a very good solution. I'd like to choose certain chores and only do those.
Parent:	O.K. Let's divide up this list. (List is divided.) We need to think up some way to see whether this solution works.
Child:	Let's try if for two weeks and see how it goes. I know this week I'm really busy with band practice, but I'll have more time next week.
Parent:	O.K., let's try it. I really feel good that we sat down and tried to work out this conflict.
Child:	Me too.

Figure 5-14   Countable versus General Behaviors or Internal States

Countable behaviors	General behaviors or internal states
made bed	was neat
set the table	helped out
hung up clothes	cleaned up
went to bed on time	cooperated
dressed self	wasn't lazy
washed dishes	tidied up
cleaned room	cleaned up
put away toys	helped out
put dishes away	was good
cleaned up spill	cleaned up
watched T.V. quietly	was quiet
finished breakfast in 1/2 hour	ate
lost 5 pounds	looked better
fed the dog	did chores
completed homework before supper	did better in school
played quietly with brother	didn't act up
drank milk	ate better
came home on time	complied
gave an "I" message	improved communication
brushed teeth	was a good girl
joined social group	increased social activities
touched others' possessions without permission	was impolite
left an area assigned to her without permission	was hyperactive

Figure 5–15 A Sample Parent–Child Contract

PROGRESS CHART

Contract:

When you have earned 25 points, you can go to a movie of your choice. You get one star (one point) for each of the tasks you complete.

Task	Sunday	Monday	Tuesday	Wednesday	Thursday	Friday	Saturday
Make bed	*						
Set the table		*	*				
Finish breakfast within 1/2 hour	*	*	*				
Feed pet rabbit by 5 p.m.		*	*				
Be in bed by 9 p.m.	*		*				
Daily total of points	3	3	4				

New contract to work on: When you have earned 20 points, you can stay up until 9:30 p.m.

Figure 5-16   Ways to Use Positive Rewards [13]

Make Positive Comments:

I like it when you play quietly (clean your room, help me without being asked, complete your homework before supper, or whatever behavior is being focused on).

You're doing a good job of losing weight (coming home on time, drinking your milk, etc.).

I liked the way you told me how you felt (cleaned up that spill without being asked, watched T.V. quietly, etc.).

I really like working (playing, talking, being) with you.

Give Physical Rewards

Reward your child after he or she has exhibited the behavior you desire to see. Choose one of the following ways to reward:

a hug	squeeze arm gently
a kiss	ruffle hair
pat on the head	pat face lightly

Remind Yourself to Reward Your Child

Make brightly colored reminder cards or signs with comments such as:

reward progress

congratulations on rewarding your child

catch your child being good

don't wait for misbehavior; reward any sign of desirable behavior

---

Figure 5–17 /// 247

Figure 5–17   Questions to Enhance Intimate Communication [18]

Area of potential conflict or communication	*Questions to ask*
1. Distance—closeness	"When do most of our arguments arise?"
	"What do our arguments tell us about our needs for greater freedom or closeness?"
	"When do I feel suffocated, deprived, or abandoned?"
	"How often and how much do I want to touch and be touched by you?"
	"How many hours can I spend with you without becoming bored, restless, or argumentative?"
	"What outside interests and involvements do I feel I need for myself?"
	"How willing are you to talk with me about these concerns I have?"
2. Centricity	"How secure do I feel in the relationship?"
	"Am I jealous of your friends or activities?"
	"Am I as important to you as you are to me?"
	"How willing are you to talk with me about these concerns?"
3. Power struggles	"How much need do I have to control what happens in the relationship?"
	"How can I express more openly with you my need to control?"
	"How can I express more openly my resentment about your dominance?"
	"How willing are you to talk with me about who is dominant?"
4. Trust formation	"How do you react when I reveal things I am sensitive about?"
	"How do you react when I am experiencing a crisis or upsetting incident?"

(continued)

Figure 5-17   (continued)

Area of potential conflict or communication	Questions to ask
	"How can I tell you about things I am sensitive about so it will be easier for you to listen to it?"
	"How can I ask you for help and be sure I'll get it when I am in a crisis?"
	"How can I talk to you about things I see you doing I don't like so you'll listen to me?"
5. Preservation of self	"How can I tell you about my need to be me in a way that you can accept?"
	"How can I tell you about my unique needs?"
	"How can I tell you in a respectful way when I feel you are violating my rights as a person?"
	"How can I tell you in a neutral way when I feel you trying to hold down my identity as a separate, unique person?"
	"How can we share household tasks so we're both satisfied?"
6. Social boundaries	"How can we decide together whom we will seek out as friends?"
	"How often will we entertain?"
	"How will we decide where we will go socially together and alone?"
	"How can I work it out with you so I can have my own social relationships?"
	"How will we decide how much time we spend with family?"
	"How can we work it out so we provide support for one another when we spend time with our own parents?"
	"How will we decide whether either of us can bring home people without prior notice?"

Figure 5-18 /// 249

Figure 5-18   Communicating about Our Sexual Experiences

Directions:

Ask yourself the questions in the left-hand column and your partner those in the right-hand one. Share the information you gain and use is to enhance your sexual relationship.

Questions to ask self	*Questions to ask my partner*
"How can I tell you when I want to make love and when I want to cuddle or hug?"	"How can I tell when you want to make love and when you want to cuddle or hug?"
"How can I help you tell me you're interested in sex so I don't feel threatened, forced, or used?"	"How can I tell you I'm interested in sex without threatening or forcing you?"
"How can we work it out when I want sex and you don't?"	"How can we work it out when you want sex and I don't?"
"What pleases me sexually?" "How can I let you know this?"	"How can I best tell you when what you do pleases me sexually?"
"How could I guide you or tell you so you know how to please me sexually?"	"How can I guide you or tell you so you know how to please me sexually?"
"What do I know about what pleases you sexually?"	"What can you tell me about what pleases you sexually?"
"What is sexual turn-off for me?"	"How can I tell you about what turns me off sexually?"
"What method of birth control do I think we should use?"	"How can I talk to you about birth control methods we plan to use in a way that enhances our sexual relationship?"
"How pleased am I with the method of birth-control we are currently using?"	
"Do I think about sex as if performance is the most important or as if pleasure is?"	"Do you think about sex as if performance is the most important or as if pleasure is?"

(continued)

Figure 5–18   (continued)

Questions to ask self	*Questions to ask my partner*
"How can I focus more of my attention on pleasure than on performance?"	"How can I help you to focus more on pleasure than on performance?"
"Do I want to introduce some new experiences or position into our sexual relationship?"	"Do you want to introduce some new experience or position into our sexual relationship?"
"What interferes with me letting go and enjoying a sexual experience?"	"What interferes with your letting go and enjoying a sexual experience?"

Figure 5-19 /// 251

Figure 5-19   Creative Visualization: Increasing Sexual Fulfillment

---

Step 1:   Use a relaxation exercise to relax deeply.

Step 2:   Focus on the problem: "How can I increase my own and my partner's sexual satisfaction?" Center your thoughts on this problem.

Step 3:   Close your eyes and visualize your partner surrounded by a halo of light and energy.

Step 4:   Project yourself into the mind and body of your partner. Allow yourself to experience being that person—what it is like to make love as your partner. Feel through your partner's body; note where you resist giving in to the experience and what helps you relax and enjoy what is happening. Experience what it is like for your partner to touch and be touched by you. Allow yourself to picture one or more sexual experiences with your partner; with each experience your sexual fulfillment increases.

Step 5:   Carry the images you conjured up of being your partner to your next sexual experience with him or her. As you begin to make love, imagine a golden light enfolding you and your partner—a light that intensifies and increases the sexual fulfillment of both of you.

Figure 5–20   Examples of Developmental or Life-Transitional Crises

---

Examples of crises people can anticipate and begin to problem-solve *before* they occur:

mid-life career changes	chronic or terminal illness
retirement	child enters or leaves school
getting married	planned entry of new family member
becoming a parent	planned surgery
divorce or separation	

Examples of unanticipated crises for which people may require additional assistance:

sudden death of a significant person	unexpected catastrophic illness
rape	sudden loss of job or status
assault	accident

Examples of crises that may or may not be anticipated and may require additional assistance:

conflicts about becoming an independent, separate person

conflicts about sexual identity

conflicts about parental versus own values

conflicts about responding to authority

conflicts about attaining self-discipline

conflicts about attaining intimacy with another person [21]

Figure 5–21   ///   253

Figure 5–21   Some Ways of Coping with Difficult Situations [22, 23]

Type of coping response	*Questions to ask*
Modifying or changing the situation	"How can I recognize the situation as the source of a problem?"
	"How can I find out what I need to know in order to eliminate the problem?"
	"From whom can I seek advice about how to modify or change the situation?"
	"How can I get in touch with what I have learned from my experiences to change the situation?"
	"How can I negotiate with important people in my life to ease the stress on me now?"
	"How can I limit others' demands on me to ease the stress on me now?"
	"What limited or short-term goals can I set to modify the situation?"
	"How can I use role playing or other rehearsal techniques to try out and choose alternate outcomes to the situation?"
Controlling the meaning of a stressful situation	"How can I compare what is happening to me now to my own (or others') experience so as to put it in perspective?"
	"How can I see the meaning of this situation as an improvement over the past?"
	"How can I view this situation as a learning experience or as a necessary part of the process of getting to my future goals?"
	"What is positive about this situation that I can focus on?"
	"What other areas of my life can I focus on so I don't pay so much attention to this stressful situation?"
	"How can I prepare for an uncertain ending to the situation by active grieving?"

(continued)

Figure 5-21 (continued)

Type of coping response	Questions to ask
	"How can I preserve the helpful parts of my relationships with others in order to help me get through this?"
	"How can I ask family, friends, or others for help, support, reassurance, or empathy?"
	"How can I de-invest myself from the situation?"
	"How can I make this stressful situation seem trivial in relation to other important areas of my life?"
	"How can I remind myself of other gratifying things in my life?"
Managing stress generated by the situation	"How can I use stress reduction techniques to relax and move through the situation?"
	"How can I look at the situation with passive forbearance?"
	"How can I accept this situation as something that is meant to be?"
	"How can I resign myself to the situation?"
	"How can I divorce myself from a sense of guilt or blame about this situation?"
	"How can I have faith about my ability to come through this?"
	"What anger ritual can I use to ventilate feeling and release my energy to deal better with the situation?"

Figure 5–22 /// 255

Figure 5–22   Examining My Life Purpose [30]

---

1. What is right with me and my life?

2. What is my special way of being that is different from anyone else?

3. What special ways am I creative?

4. How can I encourage my own way of being or creating?

5. What is blocking me from expressing myself?

6. How can I remove those blocks?

7. What is the natural direction my life should be going?

8. How can I make one small move to direct my life in that way?

9. What can I live for?

10. How can I find at least one other person who understands and accepts my view of the world?

11. How can I use creative visualization, dialogue with self, meditation, or self-hypnosis to get me in touch with what I want out of life?

12. How can I use creative visualization to get me in touch with the child within me and his or her wishes and needs so I won't have to deny them?

13. What road have I not taken that may be contributing to my unhappiness?

14. What talents do I have that I have not developed that may be contributing to my unhappiness?

15. What part of myself have I not recognized that may be contributing to my unhappiness?

16. What can I do to take a new road, develop a talent, or recognize a part of myself?

17. How can I focus more on my own (rather than on others') needs as a way to increase my wellness?

18. How do other people try to make me feel guilty or hopeless?

19. How can I anticipate these actions from others as a way to gain mastery over the situation?

20. How can I remind myself that although I can't change how people respond to me, I *can* change my response to them?

21. How can I learn to observe myself in my daily activities and begin to note whether I enjoy what I do or not?

(continued)

Figure 5–22 (continued)

22. How can I allow myself to complain and to let my frustration and anger out?

23. What ways can I use or learn to use to release anger and frustration?

24. How can I widen my life pleasures and interests so I do not focus all my energies on one relationship?

25. How can I set up checkpoints throughout my life to ask myself, "Am I doing what I want to be doing?"

26. What secret unfulfilled dreams, ambitions, or desires do I have?

27. How could I take one small step toward meeting one of them?

NOTES

1. Beatrice J. Kalisch. "What is empathy?" *American Journal of Nursing* 73, no. 9 (1973), pp. 1548-1552.
2. Barry Bricklin and Patricia Bricklin, "Psychotherapy, natural: freeing yourself and others from habits that blockade happiness." In *The Practical Encyclopedia of Natural Healing* by Mark Bricklin. Emmaus, Pa.: Rodale, 1976, p. 438.
3. Ibid., p. 444.
4. Figures 5-6-5-9 are based on ideas presented in The Boston Women's Health Book Collective. *Ourselves and Our Children: A Book by and for Parents*. New York: Random House, 1978, pp. 3-109.
5. Based on ideas presented by Hogie Wykoff. *Solving Women's Problems*. New York: Grove Press, 1977, pp. 225-228.
6. Judith F. D'Augelli and Joan M. Weener. "Training parents as mental health agents," *Community Mental Health Journal* 14, no. 1 (1978), p. 16.
7. Thomas Gordon. *P.E.T. Parent Effectiveness Training*. New York: Plume, 1975.
8. Gloria Hochman. "Drug abuse: prevention may be the best treatment of all," *Family Weekly* (October 8, 1978), p. 20.
9. R. Zucker. "Defiant youth should be target of prevention during ages 11-14," *NICAA Information and Feature Service* DHEW Publication No. (ADM) 76-151 (July 2, 1976).
10. Gordon, *P.E.T.*, p. 237.
11. Cynthia B. Hughes. "An eclectic approach to parent group education," *Nursing Clinics of North America* 12, no. 3 (1977), p. 474.
12. Ibid., pp. 474-475.
13. Based on ideas presented by Virginia Tams and Sheila Eyberg. "A group treatment program for parents." In *Behavior Modification Approaches To Parenting*, edited by Eric J. Mash, Lee C. Handy, and Leo A. Hamerlynck. New York: Brunner/Mazel, 1976, pp. 101-123.
14. M. E. Bernal. "Behavioral feedback in the modification of brat behavior," *Journal of Nervous and Mental Disease* 148 (1969), pp. 375-385.
15. Victor A. Benassi and Kathryn M. Larson. "Modification of family interaction with the child as the behavior-change agent." In Mash et al., *Behavior Modification*, pp. 331-337.
16. Nancie Mae Brown. "Rock-a-bye your baby." In *The Holistic Health Handbook* compiled by the Berkeley Holistic Health Center, Berkeley, Cal.: And/Or Press, 1978, pp. 321-323.
17. George Bach and Herb Goldberg. *Creative Aggression: The Art of Assertive Living*. New York: Avon, 1974.
18. Ibid., based on pp. 226-233.
19. Ibid., p. 507.
20. Ibid., pp. 165-190.

21. Bruce A. Baldwin. "A paradigm for the classification of emotional crises: implications for crisis intervention," *American Journal of Orthopsychiatry* 48, no. 3 (July 1978), pp. 538–551.
22. Leonard I. Pearlin and Carmi Schooler. "The structure of coping," *Journal of Health and Social Behavior* 19 (March 1978), pp. 2–21.
23. Rudolf H. Moos (ed.). *Coping with Physical Illness.* New York: Plenum Medical, 1977.
24. James J. Lynch. "Companionship, an important form of life insurance," *Prevention* (February 1978), pp. 100–104.
25. Dominick Bosco. "Friends are your best medicine," *Prevention* (September 1978), p. 158.
26. Ibid., pp. 162–163.
27. Lawrence LeShan. *You Can Fight for Your Life: Emotional Factors in the Causation of Cancer.* New York: M. Evans, 1977.
28. Ibid., pp. 32–48.
29. Ibid., p. 106.
30. Based on ideas discussed in LeShan, *You Can Fight*, pp. 110–181.

6

Fitting In

This chapter focuses on fit with the physical and social environment. As defined here, people who "fit in" with their environment have a strong sense of conservation regarding the earth's resources. Fitting in includes a deliberate effort to design and shape the home, work, and social environment as well as knowledge of how the environment shapes wellness. As with other dimensions of wellness, it is useful to remember that environmental aspects need to be considered in relation to nutrition, fitness, stress reduction, healing, caring, and responsibility. Some topics covered in this chapter are: ways of enhancing wellness, planning a life "style," and designing a living/working/playing environment.

WAYS TO ENHANCE WELLNESS

There are a number of steps you can take to improve the wellness potential of your environment. You can avoid smoke-filled, poorly-ventilated places such as bars and restaurants where smoking is permitted. You can also be more assertive about your right to clean air in airplanes, elevators, restaurants, theaters, private homes, and your workplace.

Another step you can take is to stop drinking. Alcohol is

linked to an increased risk of developing cancer of the mouth, throat, esophagus, larynx, and liver and increases the susceptibility to toxic effects of tobacco and other environmental carcinogens. Chronic use of alcohol is known to damage the liver and to impair the ability to detoxify cancer-producing substances [1].

Commonly used drugs such as depressants, narcotics, and stimulants may interact with pollutants and increase their toxic effects [2]. For this reason, *no* drugs should be taken frivolously, and alternative methods for dealing with stress should be used.

Certain food containers should be avoided. Milk and fruit juices in cans with a leaded seam can result in lead toxicity in children. Choosing food in more natural forms or in different types of containers can help avoid this source of toxicity.

Rigid polyvinyl chloride (PVC) containers have been banned because of their cancer-causing properties. However, some containers may still be on store shelves, and consumers should be on the lookout for them.

There is a wide range of drugs known to cause cancer. In fact, the most effective drugs used to treat cancer *also* cause it [3]. Since most cancers take long periods of time to develop, it may be wise for people to take one of these drugs if they already have cancer or if they are going to receive a kidney transplant, but in other cases to consider the decision carefully. Individuals need to be appraised of these risks so they can make effective decisions. "It is not . . . worth while taking carcinogenic drugs for relatively trivial conditions, such as Flagyl for (trichomonad) vaginal infections, griseofulvin for athlete's foot or for scalp infestation for ringworm, and Lindone shampoos for head lice" [4]. You can take less harmful drugs for these conditions.

Women are advised *not* to take estrogens unless menopausal symptoms are extremely debilitating and then only for a short period of time, and at a *low* dosage. Women can use methods of birth control *other than* "the pill" and refuse "morning after" pills after unprotected intercourse; instead, they can wait to see if they are pregnant and *then* have a D and C or abortion by one of the vacuum-aspiration procedures [5].

To protect against toxic substances in drinking water, you can install an activated carbon filter to your drinking water tap. These are simple to install and inexpensive, but they need to be changed every few months. Meanwhile, you can persuade your local municipal water treatment plant to install an activated carbon filtration system [6]. It is wise to disconnect (or never install) water softeners; those who drink soft drinking water are more susceptible to the development of cardiovascular disease [7], because hard water protects people from this illness. Individuals at high risk of developing cardiovascular disease (people with congestive heart disease, hypertension, renal disease, or cirrhosis of the liver) should check their home drinking water source and be sure not to drink water in other places (including hospitals) unless it, too, has been checked for its sodium level. High levels of sodium in water (or hidden sources, such as diet sodas) can cancel out the beneficial effects of a low-sodium diet.

Infants are a high-risk group, vulnerable to the toxic effects of sodium in water and milk. Cow's milk has nearly 400 percent more sodium than breast milk; infants have immature kidneys, and some may not be able to adjust to the extreme sodium levels; softened water, too, can be quite harmful to infants [8].

Those who use cosmetics need to be very selective in their choices. It is wise to avoid purchasing any products that carry the label: "Warning: The safety of this product has not been determined." Other products to avoid are those that contain known cancer-producing substances, such as 2,4-tolerenediamine or 4-methoxy-m-pherrylene-diamine used in permanent hair dyes. Any cosmetics containing yellow (dye) No. 1, Blue No. 6, and Reds No. 10, 11, 12, and 13 should not be purchased.

You need to avoid radiation exposure and should ask doctors and dentists to spell out in detail the benefits expected from possibly unnecessary x-rays. When the answer is "it's routine" or "your insurance covers it" or "for prevention," it is wise for you to pursue with questions and to make sure the x-ray is essential for the diagnosis of a serious disease or to examine an injury. Once this has been established, x-rays should *only* be done in the office of a physician who is a *specialist* in radiology or in the radiology department of a hospital; if the x-ray occurs in a radiology department, make sure the technician is *certified* (not just office trained), that modern equipment is used, that a small dose is given, and that lead shields protect all body areas not being x-rayed.

Young women should refuse x-rays to detect early breast cancer, since they may increase their chances of developing cancer; older women who have strong reason to suspect they have breast cancer can consider the risks associated with x-rays to be worthwhile. Pregnant women should consider carefully the risks—leukemia and birth defects of their child—involved in having x-rays before deciding to submit to them.

Those who are asked to have dental x-rays need to be aware that a full set need not be taken more frequently than every three to ten years, and certainly not at every routine checkup. The diagnostic information available through inspection with a dental pick is sufficient. You should also avoid extensive body x-rays given by chiropractors [9].

Individuals whose work, living, health care, or social environments are crowded may be at high risk of developing stress. Work and living environments may be rearranged to reduce interaction with others. Before subjecting yourself to additional stresses from crowding, you may want to check out available health care facilities to see how crowded they are. Social engagements can usually be planned or rearranged to suit your needs for privacy and aloneness. If environments cannot be changed physically, you may be able to use creative visualization or other stress-reduction methods to decrease the effects.

You need to avoid long hours in the sun and wear a sunscreen ointment containing para-aminobenzoic acid (PABA). Those who work outdoors can use sunblocking creams such as zinc oxide to cover sensitive areas around lips and nose. A wide sunhat and clothes that cover exposed areas are also recommended.

Those who have the ability to move out of danger areas may want to consider doing so. Those who can choose, should opt *not* to live near a chemical plant, or near a major highway or expressway. "The excess incidence of cancer in heavy industrialized counties includes women as well as men, and thus cannot be mainly due to occupational exposures" [10]. Some areas that have very high cancer mortality rates are New Jersey, New Orleans, Ohio counties near VC/PC plants, and Utah near the nuclear testing sites. As more data appear, it may be that areas such as the Love Canal, in New York, show increased cancer rates due to the concentration of toxic material.

You can inspect your home and workplace for hidden carcinogens, read labels carefully, and make sure not to purchase, use, or be around the use of the following: asbestos insulation and lining of ventilation and heating ducts, pesticides used for termite treatment and other purposes, *all* aerosols, any children's sleepwear treated with tris, or cleaning agents and solvents containing carbon tetrachloride, trichlorethylene, perchloroethylene, or benzene [11].

Your choice of work can also affect your wellness. "Workers in petrochemical, asbestos, steel, smelting, and some mining industries are recognized 'high risk' groups" [12]. Working conditions vary from the partially controlled and monitored to the totally uncontrolled, "especially in smaller nonunionized plants" [13]. The chemical industry has a history of "refusing to disclose the identity of most chemicals used in trade name products in the workplace on the grounds that these are trade secrets!" [14] People working under such conditions handle and breathe substances labeled only with letters and numbers; they need to think through the full consequences of working in an uncontrolled, high-risk industry that has a bad track record of protecting its employees. Recently, the nuclear power industry has come into question as another high-risk industry that is not well controlled and that has not protected its workers [15]. If a high-risk industry *is* chosen, it should be in a large, well-organized plant with reliable, informed union leadership. Sensitive monitors of carcinogens should be evident, and any cancer-producing substances should be handled in closed (not open) systems. Results of monitoring should be immediately available to workers, as should complete information on the names and dangers of substances being worked with. It is wise for workers to seek information about a plant's or industry's track record from an independent source [16] prior to taking a job; unfortunately, it may be difficult to obtain this kind of information, and workers need to be aware of the obstacles.

People who use arts-and-crafts material need to protect themselves from inhaling or touching harmful substances. A list of carcinogenic materials is available [17] for those involved in these activities. If there are not appropriate less lethal substitutes for the harmful substances, individuals should *only* handle them in a completely ventilated setting, with the use of a respirator, or when the process is completely enclosed.

Parents can check on the location of their children's school to make sure it is not close to harmful industries or major highways. Asbestos-spray surfaces, such as soundproofed ceilings, are dangerous and should be looked for by parents. Laboratory or physical education courses should not expose students to harmful substances or experiences. The school cafeteria and food dispensing machines are other areas to be checked out; parents are beginning to take action to ban "junk" or convenience foods [18].

To protect against the harmful effects of noise, you can begin to weigh the advantages of labor-saving but noisy devices (blenders, electric lawn mowers, etc.) versus the long-term hearing, learning, and irritability effects. You can also ask for noise reduction in your place of work. Shrubs or fences can be planted to act as sound breaks by those who live on heavily traveled streets. Ear plugs can be worn while traveling in subways or when using especially noisy equipment or transportation. Those who can move to quieter areas should be encouraged to consider it as part of a wellness program.

Acid or poisonous rain is being recognized as a growing threat to life forms. Fish are unable to survive, soil has been damaged, and the growth of plants has been retarded. Normal erosion and weathering of metal, stone buildings, and monuments has been accelerated by the increasing acidity of rain. This problem is due to the burning of fossil fuels, especially high-sulfur coal. A major problem with acid rain is that not much can be done on a local scale. Pollutants are carried aloft by prevailing winds. Increased acid in rain in one part of the country may be the result of antipollution measures taken in another; for example, the building of higher smoke stacks may result in local air clearing but will exacerbate pollution in distant places.

A related issue is that of a host of other pollutants present in the atmosphere. Small quantities of tin, arsenic, lead, and mercury may also be washed down by the rain and can be very toxic. At present, it is unclear what effect acid rain may have on human skin and hair, and what level of acidity is dangerous and over what periods of exposure [19]. For this reason, it may be prudent to wear a hat with a visor and clothes that cover the body, and/or carry an umbrella when out in the rain.

The air is filled with ions. There is a natural ratio or balance of five positive ions to four negative ones. This ratio is important. Whereas an overdose of positive ions leads to listlessness, fatigue, and irritability, an overdose of negative ions leads to peace, tranquility, concentration, and learning. On dusty or humid days there is an imbalance arising from an overdose of positive ions as the negative ions "attach themselves to particles of dust, pollution, or moisture and lose their charge" [20]. People who live and work in urban areas are especially likely to lack negative ions in the environment. Automobiles, pollution, smoking, clothes and furniture made of synthetic fibers, new types of building materials, modern transportation, and central heating and cooling systems in "hermetically sealed high-rise office buildings—all of these are part of man-made environments that have too few ions of both kinds for healthy, normal life" [21].

Negative ions can be increased by living and working in environments that are not synthetic, that do not have central air conditioning and heating, and that are not hermetically sealed. You can make an effort to purchase and wear natural fibers such as cotton, wool, linen, leather, and silk. If you have a choice of office, job, or workspace, choose those that are near trees, fountains, water, and plants. People who must work and live in sealed-in environments can make an effort during lunch to go outdoors to an open environment such as a park, where there are trees and negative ions, or to a fountain or lake. Those who are unable to do any of these can spray their work area with water; buy (or suggest management provide) trees and plants for the work area; drive with a window slightly open (rather than with all windows closed and the vents open or air conditioning on); breathe in deeply several times a day through the left nostril—this provides negatively ionized air; visit large water fountains, water falls, or the ocean whenever possible. In addition people can clean less frequently; negative ions are attracted to dust. Also, people who have wall-to-wall carpeting should walk on it in their stockinged feet; the friction built up from shoes and synthetic carpets creates an overabundance of positive ions [22]. As a last resort, individuals can buy (or petition management to buy) a negative ion generator. These generators are beginning to be used by business firms to enhance the attention span and learning of business trainees [23] and in medicine to enhance recovery of people who have had surgery, delivered a baby, suffered from severe burns, have hay fever, asthma, or anxiety neurosis [24]. Lacking of any of these choices, people can choose vacations where they have access to the sea, water falls, mountains or hilly areas, and where there is abundant sunshine and clear air.

Natural light appears to be a nutrient needed by the body. People who wear glasses or contact lenses all day, who wear sunglasses when outside, who remain inside a car or building from sun-up to sunset, or who work all day under fluorescent lights are apt to be deficient in natural light. Artificial light is deficient in certain constituents of full-spectrum light and is an inferior type of light.

Natural light strikes the retina of the eye, stimulates the optic nerve, and sends impulses to the hypothalamus (a part of the brain that influences emotion). Most studies about the effects of light on growth and on the secretion of endocrine organs have been done on animals, but there have been noticeable differences in the size of their spleens, hearts, and reproductive organs. One study originally done in Russia and replicated in the United States demonstrated that school children who had low levels of ultraviolet light added to the school lighting system were less hyperactive, had higher grades, and grew faster. Another study revealed that students had less fatigue and better visual acuity when using full-spectrum rather than fluorescent lighting. In yet another research venture, hamsters who had slow-acting tumor transplants injected took significantly longer to develop tumors in natural light than they did in fluorescent light environments [25].

People who want to minimize the effect of polluted light can do a number of things. One of them is to walk to work, go outdoors into the light at noon, and to wait for friends or associates outside buildings during the day rather than in the lobby. It is not important to be in the sunlight, what is important is to be in the natural, full-spectrum light. Another thing to do is never to wear sunglasses unless it is absolutely necessary. Those who wear corrective glasses can consider investing in lenses that absorb the light uniformly. These full-spectrum lenses can be ordered by an optometrist or opthalmologist. Another measure is to install full-spectrum, sun-simulating Vita-Lites in key spots at home and work. Another suggestion is to purchase a sunlamp and lie under it several times a week for short periods of time, being careful not to become overexposed. Ultraviolet light is believed to stimulate enzyme reactions, increase the activity of the endocrine system, and increases immunological or protective body responses. In Russia, daily low exposures of ultraviolet light are used to treat coal miners who have black lung. The U.S. Navy uses it with submarine personnel; there has been less illness among treated crewmen, and reports of emotional benefit [26]. The benefits of ultraviolet light are just beginning to be known.

Figure 6-1 summarizes harmful factors in the environment [27–38]. Figure 6-2 gives important information about protection from these harmful aspects of our environment. Although each kind of pollution has potential for affecting each person, each individual has his or her own unique genetic composition and threshold of sensitivity. For this reason, it may be useful to use Diamond's muscle test (see Chapter 2) to assess which substances are potentially toxic, based on the client's muscle weakness or strength. Dr. Diamond suggests that people who test weak can strengthen their thymus by thumping it [39].

Although there is some information available about the environment and its effect on wellness, there is still much to be learned. Most is known about substances that can cause cancer. Yet even here wide gaps in knowledge are evident. Research on the environmental causes of cancer is difficult, but the major problems are *not* the research difficulty. Rather, lags in this area are due to the fact that *less than 15 percent* of all federal funds for cancer research are being spent on environmental research, *despite* the fact that the National Cancer Institute estimates that 90 percent of all cancer is environmentally caused. Another major problem is that businesses are the major polluters, and they often have a financial interest in products that pollute. It is not even the efforts to slow down and impede regulation of hazardous substances that is the major problem, but the presentation of fraudulent data [40]:

> It now appears that a major portion of the data upon which the safety of pesticides was judged was, in fact, fraudulent. It may well turn out that levels of pesticides and other chemicals previously thought to be safe are not safe at all.

These are the kinds of problems for which it is difficult to take protection measures except in terms of people taking actions to monitor the medical-industrial-governmental complex. These issues will be addressed in greater depth in Chapter 7.

PLANNING AN ENVIRONMENTALLY SOUND LIFE STYLE

Life styles either affirm or deny other efforts toward wellness. There are many environmental problems to worry about and to work to change. But, those who are interested in enhancing their own (and others') wellness also do their own part to conserve available resources. Some ways to do this are to try to live in places where dangerous substances are not in the air and water and to buy foods that are lower on the food chain and thus less susceptible to environmental pollution. People who do not already enjoy such foods as rice, beans, wheat, barley, oats, and soybeans can begin to develop a taste for them. These foods require less energy to produce and are less polluted.

You can conserve energy by turning off lights and machines that require power when they are not in use and by setting aside periods of time (and gradually increasing these periods) when high-energy vehicles or machines are not used at all. You need to begin to question whether time-saving machines and gadgets are really worth the energy they consume. Ensuring your home is well-insulated will conserve energy and money. Walking not only saves energy but is a good measure for relieving stress and toning the body. Consider avoiding disposable and processed products and increasing the use of recycled items. Even city-bound people can plant a herb garden and some tomato plants in a pot; garden work is both tension-relieving and energy-saving. Instead of buying fertilizer, save uncooked fresh vegetable and fruit ends, skins, and so forth and "grow" your own compost. Avoid fast food chains since they are high-energy consumers.

Those who smoke can look for a stop-smoking program, or take up jogging. Joggers often report that they stop smoking once they begin to feel the benefits from this form of exercise. Those who do not smoke can begin to assert themselves with others who do. (See Figure 6–3.)

Energy resources are *not* infinite. Because this is so, many futurists suggest that the best way to conserve resources is to have fewer children. There are many unwanted infants, tots, and older children, especially with learning disabilities, handicaps, and other disadvantages. People who wish to have a personal parenting experience can consider adopting those already born.

DESIGNING A LIVING/WORKING/PLAYING ENVIRONMENT

There may be a wide range of options for designing or shaping an environment. Despite limitations, some options are open to all people. The first step to take is to assess various aspects of the environment for fit, stress, and liking. Some questions to ask appear in Figures 6-4 to 6-6.

Most of the questions appearing in Figure 6-4 relate to information presented earlier in this chapter. Figure 6-5 offers some new information. Wellness in the work environment may well be related to the quality of working life. Walton [41] has proposed eight categories for analyzing this aspect of wellness: adequate and fair compensation; safe and healthy working conditions; immediate opportunity to use and develop human capacities; future opportunity for continued growth and security; social integration in the work organization; constitutionalism in the work organization; work and the total life space; and, the social relevance of work.

Adequacy of pay is harder to assess than fairness. If workers think they are receiving compensation that is in line with their training and education, entails appropriate responsibility, and makes up for noxious working conditions, they are apt to view their pay as adequate. Safe and healthy working conditions include reasonable hours with premium pay for overtime, physical working conditions that minimize the chance of injury or illness and maximize comfort, and age limits on work potentially detrimental to specific age groups. Although safe and healthy working conditions comprise only one category of quality of work, it seems to be important. An eight-year study has revealed that 78 percent of the workers surveyed said their jobs exposed them to at least one health or safety hazard, including air pollution, fire or safety hazards, noise, and dangerous chemicals [42]. Thus, a large percentage of workers surveyed cannot be attaining a high level of wellness in the work area.

Another aspect of the quality of work—an opportunity to use and develop capacities—includes doing a whole (not fragmented) task, obtaining information that puts one's job in the larger perspective of the organization, planning as well as implementing tasks, using a wide range of skills and abilities, and job autonomy, as well as opportunities to maintain and expand capabilities, to use expanded or newly acquired knowledge and skills on the job, and advancement opportunities. Social integration in the workplace includes, among others, freedom from prejudice, egalitarianism, mobility, support from work groups, a sense of community, and interpersonal openness. The category of constitutionalism includes the right to personal privacy regarding off-the-job behavior, to disagree with superiors without fear of reprisal, to equal treatment, and to due process. A major element of work and the total life space that determines wellness is the extent of the positive or negative effect of the job on workers' relationships with their families. When work requirements take up leisure and family time on a regular basis, an imbalance is likely to occur. A final aspect of the quality of work is related to workers' perceptions of the organization's social responsibility in terms of its products, waste disposal, marketing techniques, employment practices, relations to underdeveloped countries, and participation in political campaigns [43].

Tension can burn up energy that could be used in productive work. Energy is lost when workers feel someone is looking over their shoulder and pressuring them, or that internal or external time schedules lead to additional stress, when work is boring, uncomfortable, under- or overstimulating, when working conditions or the physical environment is crowded or disorganized, or when a great deal of time is used gossiping, flirting, or complaining.

Another aspect to survey when discussing the work environment is the ability to be assertive and to be accepted—though not necessarily with—when being assertive. Some important skills needed for this are of planning short- and long-term goals, saying no to illegitimate requests, stopping requests, completing work in a reasonable time frame, persisting in achieving change, owning up to mistakes, asking for help, completing unpleasant tasks, structuring work to be rewarding, and taking a reasonable risk. Being able to do each of these in a confident and comfortable manner can enhance work.

Figure 6-6 deals with a more elusive aspect, play. Many adults think only children play, yet both children and adults need play, although for different reasons. For children, play is serious stuff— a way of learning about the world. For adults, play is a voluntary activity; one cannot be ordered to play. This quality of freedom marks play off from tasks. It is done during leisure in "free time." Although play has a "let's pretend" quality, this does not prevent it from being experienced in the utmost seriousness. Play provides an interlude, a release from the drudgery and boredom of the usual pattern of things. Play is also time-limited; it may erupt in a moment of joy, intimacy, or stress into teasing, or love-play, or a more ordered form such as chess or checkers. Whichever form it takes, it begins, and at a certain point it is over [44]. Play provides a needed contrast from the bondage and anxieties of work and life; both work and play are necessary for a balanced state of wellness.

People may be at the height of their humanness when they play. A childlike (but not childish) sense of autonomy, spontaneity, and intimacy can occur when people allow their "child" [45] or the playful part of themselves to emerge. All adults have playful aspects of themselves, learned in childhood but often suppressed by the stern "parent" parts of themselves. Leisure and play is especially difficult for Americans who have been raised to view work as "good" and idleness as "bad" [46]. It is useful to get away from these judgmental categories and view leisure as an attitude or condition during which activities are engaged in merely for the purpose of engaging in them. This kind of view makes the process more important than the product; for example, the enjoyment of going fishing is there in and of itself, regardless of how many fish are caught. People who are unable to enjoy their leisure as a process (rather than as a competitive event) are not apt to benefit as much from the stress-reducing benefits as others who relax and enjoy the activity.

Figure 6-1 Harmful Factors in the Environment [28-39]

Factors	Dangers
Consumer products	inconsistent testing, labeling, and dispersal of information
Fabrics and textiles	carcinogenic flame retardants added to fabric and textiles
Prescribed drugs	pharmaceutical industry and prescribing physicians do not make full information available to clients
	depressants, narcotics, and stimulants may interact with pollutants to increase their toxic effect

Figure 6-1 /// 271

Prescribed drugs *(continued)*	estrogens increase risk of breast and other cancers in self and offspring, coronary heart disease, hypertension, stroke, gallbladder disease
Alcohol	promotes or enhances the carcinogenic effects of other agents in the environment
Cigarettes	lung and possibly other cancers
	interferes with cleansing and healing mechanisms of the lung
	increased tar, carbon monoxide, nicotine, and nitrosamine inhalation of the nonsmoker through exposure to harmful sidestream smoke
	damage to lung tissue
	increased risk of dying from lung cancer due to exposure to other pollutants such as asbestos
	increased risk of stroke and heart attacks in women who take estrogens
	children of smokers have a higher rate of pneumonia and bronchitis
Pesticides	fraudulent test results and withholding of findings
	resistance of insects to inorganic pesticides and evolution of newer, possibly more lethal species
	deaths and hospitalization of workers exposed to pesticides
	deaths and contamination of animals and fish
	unknown effects due to contamination of soil, surface (including drinking) water, dairy products, and breast milk
	cancer of the liver
The workplace and its emissions	ineffective measures of harmful emissions and inadequate protection of workers

(continued)

Figure 6–1   (continued)

Factors	*Dangers*
Asbestos	increased rate of lung cancers and probably all cancers as well as asbestosis for workers in asbestos plants
Polyvinyl chloride and vinyl chloride	increased rate for cancer of the liver, kidney, brain, and lung arthritis, clubbing of fingers and toes, spasms of blood vessels, liver damage, chronic lung disease, chronic gastritis, dizziness, disorientation, headaches, painful bone changes for workers in PVC/VC plants and a type of asthma in people who wrap meat using hot wires or cool rods to cut and seal plastic wrappings
Dangerous plant emissions	unknown risk to people living in the vicinity of asbestos, rubber, chemical, plastic, PVC/VC steel, smelting and some mining operations
Bischloromethylether	increased risk of lung cancer for textile workers who use formaldehyde in making permanent press fabrics and use acid wash
Crowding	high stress; possibly violence and inability to do constructive work
Benzene	toxic bone marrow effects for those exposed to emissions from coke ovens, dye removers, solvents, photoetching dyes, silkscreen washes, petrochemical refineries, petrochemical plants, gasoline pumps at gas stations, auto exhaust, repair cement, carburetor cleaners, paint and wood strippers; unknown toxic effects to workers in solvent industries
Illegal dumping of toxic wastes	depends on the waste

Figure 6–1 /// 273

Factors	Dangers
Radiation	effects are additive; effects of low-level radiation create immediate changes in cell structure and long-term exposure increases risk of cancers; risk increases as level of radiation increases; safe levels are in question at present, and monitoring devices are crude
Noise	hearing loss, elevated blood pressure, tension, nervousness, imbalance in the fluid and electrolytes as well as the hormonal balance of the reproductive system
Ions	increase in positive ionization from automobiles, smoking, synthetic clothes, new types of building materials, modern transportation, and central heating and cooling systems resulting in listlessness, fatigue, irritability, and inability to concentrate
Light	fluorescent and less-than-full-spectrum light may retard growth and have negative effects on behavior
High voltage lines	unknown biological effects
Acid rain	deaths of fish, damage to soil and plant growth, acceleration of weathering, unclear effects to human skin and hair

*For further explanation of risks in the workplace see: P. Cole and M. B. Goldman, Occupation (Chapter 11) in J. F. Fraumeni, Jr., ed. *Persons at High Risk of Cancer,* New York: Academic Press, 1975, pp. 167–184.

For further information on consumer products see: Samuel S. Epstein, *The Politics of Cancer,* San Francisco: Sierra Club, 1978.

For further information on environmental pollutants see: Edward J. Calabrese, *Pollutants and High Risk Groups,* New York: Wiley, 1978.

Figure 6-2   Protection from Harmful Aspects of the Environment

Harmful substances/occurrences	High-risk groups	Protective measures
Tar, carbon monoxide, nicotine, and nitrosamines of cigarette smoke	people with cardiovascular and respiratory illnesses; unborn children	stop smoking; stay away from areas where others smoke; increase Vitamin C, A
Alcohol	people who smoke	stop drinking
Nitrosamines		stop eating cured meats and cheeses; stop smoking or being near smokers; do not live near plants that manufacture plastics or rubber; ban nitrite as a food preservative; take additional Vitamin C and E
Asbestos	workers in plants producing asbestos or asbestos products; people who use consumer products containing asbestos; hobbyists and artists using plasterboard spackle; children in schools where asbestos is used	demand informed consent regarding dangers and surveillance program for former asbestos workers; read product labels carefully; parents can inspect schools for asbestos and enlist help of PTA or local legislator

Cans with leaded seams	children	choose food packaged in other types of containers; increase intake of calcium, iron, phosphorus, protein, and Vitamins A, D, C
Ozone	people with asthma, chronic respiratory and heart disease black persons with G-6-PD deficiency	increase intake of Vitamin A, C, E, selenium
Benzene	artists, hobbyists, workers in industry	increase intake of Vitamin C; do not use products containing Benzene
Fluoridated water	people who eat large amounts of protein, calcium, Vitamin D, and alcohol; those over age 50	increase magnesium intake
Manganese dust	miners with iron deficiencies	increase iron intake
Cadmium	pregnant women, some artists and hobbyists	increase selenium and zinc intake; correct any iron deficiencies
Prescribed drugs	people receiving synthetic hormones, radiosotopes; immuno-suppressive drugs, cytotoxic drugs, arsenic, phenacetin containing drugs, coal tar ointments	be sure you are appraised of all risks before deciding to submit to the treatment

Figure 6-2 (continued)

Harmful substances/occurrences	High-risk groups	Protective measures
Hair dyes	people who dye their hair	read labels carefully;
		write to manufacturers for information; medium and dark-haired people can use henna; streaking, tipping, or frosting are safer and should be used instead of dyes; use natural lighteners such as lemon juice or chamomile tea
Estrogens	sexually active women	use other forms of birth control;
		take additional magnesium if on "the pill";
		take iodine or kelp
	women who have been raped	refuse "morning-after" pill; have D & C or abortion if pregnant
	menopausal women	try Vitamin E for debilitating symptoms; take estrogens only in low doses for short periods of time; take kelp
Various pollutants in drinking	depends on pollutant	install activated carbon filter on drinking water tap

Soft water	people with congestive heart disease, hypertension, renal disease, cirrhosis of the liver, infants	disconnect or never install water softener; check drinking water source for sodium content; consider breast-feeding infants
Cosmetics	unknown	avoid purchasing any products carrying warning labels 2, 4-toluene-diamine or 4 methoxy-in-phenylene-diamine, Yellow #1, Blue #6, and Reds #10–#13
Radiation; x-rays	young women who suspect breast cancer, pregnant women, children, unborn fetuses	avoid unnecessary x-rays; insist on hearing in detail the benefits expected from radiation exposure; have x-rays done only by a specialist or in a radiology department using modern equipment, small doses, and adequate body shields; take kelp, pectin, bioflavonoids, pantothenic acid, Vitamin B_3, C, and bee pollen
Sun	outdoor workers and sunbathers	wear sunscreen (PABA) and protective clothing; avoid long hours in the sun if possible
Nuclear radiation emissions	people closest to emissions, children, unborn fetuses, those who have had massive x-rays	increase intake of Vitamin C, kelp, pectin, or dolomite; increase intake of pantothenic acid, Vitamin B_3, and bee pollen

Figure 6-2 (continued)

Harmful substances/occurrences	High-risk groups	Protective measures
Accidents	same	same; in addition: stay indoors when radioactive plume is passing over; evacuate if pregnant or a child to outside 30-mile range; insist reactors have iodine filters installed have several days' supply of food and water on hand have potassium iodide on hand (to protect against cancer of the thyroid)
Crowding	people with ethnic or personally defined needs for space that are not met	redesign environment or use stress-reduction technique to decrease crowding effects

Sources: Edward J. Calabrese, *Pollutants and High Risk Groups*, New York: Wiley, 1978.
Samuel S. Epstein, *The Politics of Cancer*, San Francisco: Sierra Club, 1978.
Teach-in on Nuclear Power from Riverside Church, WBAI, May 5, 1979.

Figure 6-3 /// 279

Figure 6-3   Model Response for Smoking Assertion

Smoker:	"You don't mind if I smoke, do you?"
Nonsmoker:	"Yes, I do."
Smoker:	Ignores comment and lights up.
Nonsmoker:	"I do mind if you smoke."
Smoker:	"Hey, hey, don't get excited."
Nonsmoker:	"I'm not excited, but I am concerned about my health. Smoke from others' cigarettes is bad for my health."
Smoker:	"Well, leave then. I'm smoking."
Nonsmoker:	"We need to get this work done, but I maintain my right to breathe clean air."
Smoker:	"So, what are we going to do?"
Nonsmoker:	"I suggest we finish up this work and then I'll leave."
Smoker:	"I need a cigarette now."
Nonsmoker:	"Do you want to take a break first?"
Smoker:	"No, no. I want to get this work done."

Figure 6–4   Assessing My Living Environment

		Yes	No	*Would like to change this*
1.	I think the air in my neighborhood is fresh and clean and invigorating	......	......	......
2.	The place where I live is stressful to me	......	......	......
3.	I make sure I purchase safe consumer products	......	......	......
4.	My work space at home is organized the way I like it	......	......	......
5.	My sleep space is organized the way I like it	......	......	......
6.	My eating space is organized to enhance my eating pleasure	......	......	......
7.	I organize my living environment to enhance my wellness	......	......	......
8.	I reduce the noise level in my living environment whenever I can	......	......	......
9.	I make sure I receive adequate exposure to full-spectrum light	......	......	......
10.	I avoid exposure to microwave sources	......	......	......
11.	I keep track of the number and exposure of x-rays I get	......	......	......
12.	I question practitioners before accepting an x-ray	......	......	......
13.	I only accept x-rays when I am protected with body shielding and the technician is certified	......	......	......
14.	My home environment provides negative ions	......	......	......
15.	I wear as many natural-fabric clothes as I can	......	......	......

Figure 6-4 /// 281

		Yes	No	*Would like to change this*
16.	I take note of those synthetic fabrics in clothes or furnishings that seem to affect me adversely	......	......	......
17.	I make sure I stay away from high-voltage lines	......	......	......
18.	I eat low on the food chain	......	......	......
19.	I avoid smoking and people who smoke	......	......	......
20.	I avoid drinking alcoholic beverages	......	......	......
21.	I make sure I know the *exact* effects of any medication I take	......	......	......
22.	I read labels of all consumer products I buy and am aware of any harmful ingredients	......	......	......
23.	I avoid products in cans with leaded seams	......	......	......
24.	I know about the location of toxic wastes near my home	......	......	......
25.	I am aware of the possible harmful effects of rain	......	......	......
26.	I stay away from fatty foods, and I am aware of foods that have high concentrations of pollutants	......	......	......
27.	I have stopped eating highly processed junk foods	......	......	......
28.	I use an activated charcoal filter on my drinking water tap *or* know my community water source uses one	......	......	......

(continued)

Figure 6–4   (continued)

		Yes	No	Would like to change this
29.	I avoid using water softeners	......	......	......
30.	I avoid long hours in the sun or wear protective clothing and an effective sunscreen ointment	......	......	......
31.	I am aware of the location of chemical plants, refineries, asbestos plants, metal mining, or processing plants, and major highways near my home	......	......	......
32.	I inspect my home regularly for hidden carcinogens	......	......	......
33.	I avoid wearing sunglasses	......	......	......
34.	I use Diamond's muscle test to assess what things in my environment are stressful to me	......	......	......
35.	There are sufficient plants, flowers, and trees in my environment	......	......	......
36.	I turn off lights I am not using	......	......	......
37.	I try to use energy-consuming machines less often	......	......	......
38.	I avoid using disposable and highly processed products	......	......	......
39.	I grow some of my own food	......	......	......
40.	I find opportunities to listen to and enjoy the natural outdoor sounds— birds singing, rain falling, water falling, etc.	......	......	......

Figure 6-4 /// 283

		Yes	No	*Would like to change this*
41.	I find opportunities to smell and to enjoy natural outdoor smells— freshly mown hay or grass, flowers, etc.	......	......	......
42.	My life allows me chances to give and take affection	......	......	......
43.	The place I live allows me the opportunity to be near friends and support networks	......	......	......
44.	My living environment affords me chances for leisure activity	......	......	......
45.	I am free from bodily harm in my neighborhood	......	......	......
46.	My neighborhood reinforces my attempts to enhance my wellness	......	......	......
47.	My living environment provides positive feedback to me on my accomplishments	......	......	......
48.	I sense I have a bad fit with my living environment because I do not feel peaceful and relaxed there	......	......	......

Figure 6–5   Assessing My Work Environment

		Yes	No	Would like to change this
1.	The air in my work environment is free from smoke and harmful pollutants	......	......	......
2.	I work with materials that are safe *or* my employer provides enclosed, safe ways to work with materials	......	......	......
3.	I am aware of the nature and possible harmful effects of the materials I work with	......	......	......
4.	I try to avoid some of the positive ion effects in my work-place	......	......	......
5.	The noise level at work is low and/or I wear protective ear coverings	......	......	......
6.	I take steps to increase my exposure to full-spectrum light	......	......	......
7.	If I am in a high-risk (for cancer) job, I am aware of it	......	......	......
8.	I go outside during lunch break and increase my exposure to full-spectrum light and negative ions	......	......	......
9.	I am interested in the work I do	......	......	......
10.	I have just the right amount of work to do	......	......	......
11.	There is just enough change in my work and working conditions to make it interesting	......	......	......
12.	My boss is open to ideas from me and willing to communicate openly	......	......	......

Figure 6-5 /// 285

		Yes	No	*Would like to* *change this*
13.	I receive support from my superiors and coworkers	......	......	......
14.	I spend little work time gossiping, flirting, and complaining	......	......	......
15.	I have a say in decisions that affect me	......	......	......
16.	I find ways to increase my satisfaction at work	......	......	......
17.	My work is meaningful to me	......	......	......
18.	I work up to my full capacity	......	......	......
19.	I work at regular hours that are comfortable for me	......	......	......
20.	I know exactly what is expected of me and my work	......	......	......
21.	I have interactions with just the right number of people each day	......	......	......
22.	I have sufficient personal work space to concentrate and feel comfortable	......	......	......
23.	My work materials are (and remain) in an order that works well for me	......	......	......
24.	My work allows me to express myself and develop my potential	......	......	......
25.	I sense I have a good fit with my work environment because I feel energetic and productive	......	......	......
26.	I bring personal touches or possessions to my work place to make it seem more like my space	......	......	......
27.	My work allows me to distribute my body weight evenly and reduce additional strain to my body	......	......	......

(continued)

Figure 6–5 (continued)

		Yes	No	*Would like to change this*
28.	I plan several short breaks for myself where I breathe deeply and relax my whole body on exhalation	......	......	......
29.	I think that the salary I receive is right for the work I do	......	......	......
30.	My work allows me to grow and develop as a person	......	......	......
31.	People I work with seem to value me and my work	......	......	......
32.	My work affords me the possibility of planning short- and long-term goals	......	......	......
33.	I am able to clearly tell coworkers what I expect from them and find out what they expect from me	......	......	......
34.	I can say no to illegitimate work requests	......	......	......
35.	I can stop others from interrupting me so I can complete my work in a reasonable time frame	......	......	......
36.	I can persist when there is some aspect of my work that is bothersome and that I want changed	......	......	......
37.	I can own up to my mistakes or errors without shifting the blame or overapologizing	......	......	......
38.	I can ask for assistance in completing tasks when I need help and be pretty sure I'll get it	......	......	......
39.	I plan a way to complete unpleasant work tasks	......	......	......

Figure 6-5 /// 287

		Yes	No	*Would like to change this*
40.	I structure my work to reward myself	......	......	......
41.	I can take a reasonable risk without feeling unduly anxious or without encountering unreasonable retaliation	......	......	......
42.	I pace my work at a rate that feels comfortable to me	......	......	......
43.	My work environment is free from prejudice of all kinds	......	......	......
44.	There is a sense of community or shared purpose among the workers	......	......	......
45.	My work allows me privacy about my off-the-job behavior	......	......	......
46.	I am free to disagree with superiors without fear of reprisal	......	......	......
47.	I am treated equitably in terms of compensation, rewards, and job security	......	......	......
48.	My work environment provides me with due process in work-related matters	......	......	......
49.	My work is balanced in relation to my needs for leisure and time with family and friends	......	......	......
50.	My work provides me with a sense of continuity and stability	......	......	......
51.	My work organization is socially responsible in its products, waste disposal, marketing techniques, employment practices, relationships with underdeveloped countries, and its participation in political campaigns	......	......	......
52.	Supervision of my work is provided in a helpful, growth-enhancing way	......	......	......

Figure 6-6   Assessing My Play Environment

		Yes	No	Would like to change this
1.	I find places to spend my leisure time where the air is fresh and clean and invigorating	......	......	......
2.	I organize my leisure activities to enhance my wellness	......	......	......
3.	I reduce the noise level of or near my leisure activities	......	......	......
4.	I stay away from movies, television, or leisure activities that upset me and increase my stress level	......	......	......
5.	I participate in leisure activities that allow me to "get turned on," play, have fun, and be spontaneous	......	......	......
6.	I allow myself to be outrageous, wild, or passionate during my "play" times	......	......	......
7.	My play times allow me to escape from habit and open up new, unrevealed parts of myself	......	......	......
8.	I allow myself to be uninhibited and fun-loving during my leisure time	......	......	......
9.	I give myself up to the here-and-now and thoroughly enjoy my leisure time	......	......	......
10.	I choose companions for my leisure	......	......	......
11.	I believe in my ability to fully enjoy my leisure time	......	......	......
12.	I am able to balance my leisure time among feeling, knowing, and doing	......	......	......
13.	I take a vacation at least once a year	......	......	......

Figure 6–6 /// 289

		Yes	No	*Would like to change this*
14.	I spend some of my leisure time alone, doing things I like	......	......	......
15.	I spend some of my leisure time with other people whose company I enjoy	......	......	......
16.	I enjoy the process of leisure activities and am not so concerned with their outcome	......	......	......
17.	My leisure and play times provide a needed refreshment from my usual activities	......	......	......
18.	I have a balance between leisure and work time	......	......	......

(continued)

NOTES

1. Edward J. Calabrese. *Pollutants and High-Risk Groups*. New York: Wiley, 1978, pp. 147-148.
2. Ibid., p. 149.
3. R. Hoover and J. F. Fraumeni, Jr. "Drugs." In *Persons at High Risk of Cancer*, edited by J. F. Fraumeni, Jr. New York: Academic Press, 1975, pp. 185-200.
4. Samuel S. Epstein. *The Politics of Cancer*. San Francisco: Sierra Club, 1978, p. 445.
5. Ibid.
6. Ibid., p. 444.
7. Calabrese, *Pollutants*, pp. 126-127.
8. Ibid., pp. 127-128.
9. Epstein, *Politics*, pp. 447-449.
10. Ibid., pp. 450-451.
11. Ibid., pp. 452-454.
12. Ibid., p. 454.
13. Ibid., p. 455.
14. Ibid.
15. "Trial nears an end in Silkwood death," *New York Times*, May 6, 1979, p. 49.
16. Epstein, *Politics*, pp. 454-456.
17. Ibid., p. 457, Table 11.1.
18. Ibid., pp. 456-458.
19. Albert Rosenfield. "Forecast: poisonous rain," *Saturday Review* (September 2, 1978), pp. 16-17.
20. Fred Soyka, *The Ion Effect*. New York: Bantam, 1977, p. 21.
21. Ibid., p. 82.
22. Soyka, *Ion Effect*, pp. 81-105 and 116-121; John Diamond. *BK Behavioral Kinesiology*, New York: Harper & Row, 1979, p. 83.
23. "Can 'air vitamins' revitalize your trainees?" *Training* 15, no. 9 (1978), p. 94.
24. Soyka, *Ion Effect*, pp. 58-105.
25. Catherine Houck. "Caution: artificial light may be hazardous to your health," *New York Magazine* (December 1978).
26. Ibid., p. 34.
27. International Agency for Research on Cancer. *Sex Hormones. Monograph on the Evaluation of Carcinogenic Chemicals to Man* 6, Lyon, France, 1974.
28. W. J. Diekmann et al. "Does the administration of Diethylstilbestrol during pregnancy have any therapeutic value?" *American Journal of Obstetrics and Gynecology* 66 (1953), pp. 1062-1081.
29. M. Bibbo et al. "Follow-up study of male and female offspring of DES-exposed mothers," *Journal of The American College of Obstetrics and Gynecology* 49 (1977), pp. 1-8.

30. "Mortality associated with the pill," *Lancet* 2 (1977), pp. 747-748.
31. Royal College of General Practitioners' Oral Contraception Study. "Mortality among oral contraceptive users," *Lancet* 2 (1977), p. 727.
32. M. P. Vessey, K. McPherson, and B. Johnson. "Mortality among women participating in the Oxford family planning association contraceptive study," *Lancet* 2 (1977), p. 731.
33. International Agency for Research on Cancer. *Some organo-chlorine pesticides. IARC Monographs on the Evaluation of Carcinogenic Risk of Chemicals to Man* 5, Lyon, France, 1974.
34. D. Pimental. *Ecological effects of pesticides on non-target species.* Washington, D.C.: Office of Science and Technology, June, 1971.
35. U. Saffiotti and J. K. Wagoner, eds. *Occupational Carcinogenesis. Annals of the New York Academy of Sciences* 271, New York, 1976.
36. W. J. Nicholson, "Occupational and environmental standards for asbestos and their relation to human disease." In *Origins of Human Cancer*, vol. 4, edited by H. Hiatt, J. D. Watson, and J. A. Winsten. Cold Spring Harbor Laboratory, 1977, pp. 1785-1796.
37. P. F. Infante. "Oncogenic and mutagenic risks in communities with PVC production facilities." In Saffiotti and Wagoner, *Occupational Carcinogenesis*, pp. 49-57.
38. S. J. Mara and S. S. Lee. *Human exposures to atmospheric benzene.* Center for Resource and Environmental Systems Studies Report 30, Stanford, Calif.: Stanford Research Institute, 1977.
39. John Diamond. *BK Behavioral Kinesiology.* New York: Harper & Row, 1979, pp. 22 and 74.
40. Donald M. Vickery. *Life Plan for Your Health.* Reading, Mass.: Addison-Wesley, 1978, pp. 189-190.
41. Richard E. Walton. "Quality of working life: what is it?" *Sloan Management Review* 15 (Fall 1973), pp. 11-21.
42 Robert P. Quinn and Grahm L. Staines. "Job satisfaction has decreased," *Institute of Social Research Newsletter* University of Michigan (Spring 1979), pp. 10-11.
43. Walton, *Quality of Working Life*, pp. 11-21.
44. J. Huizinga. "Play and contest as civilizing functions." In *Play: Its Role in Development and Evolution*, edited by Jerome S. Bruner, Alison Jolly, and Kathy Sylva. New York: Basic Books, 1976, pp. 675-687.
45. This is Eric Berne's theory that at any given moment a person is acting in one of three distinct ways: as Parent, Adult, or Child. For further comments see: Eric Berne. *Games People Play.* New York: Grove Press, 1964.
46. Thomas F. Green. *Work, Leisure, and the American Schools.* New York: Random House, 1968, pp. 57-58.

7

Being Responsible

This chapter examines one of the forces that affect responsibility for wellness, namely beliefs, and gives suggestions for taking more responsibility in ending smoking, handling emergencies, when and how to seek and choose a health care practitioner, peer and group help, relation to drugs you take, and projects to get involved in to increase responsibility.

Responsibility is a dimension that interweaves with all other dimensions. In fact, this interweaving is evident in the preceding chapters; the issue of responsibility is mentioned throughout. This chapter could have as easily been presented as the introductory instead of the final chapter. Responsibility closes the circle of wellness dimensions.

BELIEFS AND RESPONSIBILITY

Your beliefs about wellness can influence the degree of responsibility you take. People seem to be divided into two groups: those who attribute what happens to them to external forces, and those who believe that what happens to them is due to their own actions or their own permanent characteristics. Rotter [1] refers to these centers of *perceived* control as external control and internal control. People who believe that their wellness is out of their control usually perceive what happens to them as due to luck, chance, fate, heredity, powerful others, or as unpredictable. People who believe their wellness is within their control perceive what happens to them as due to their own behavior or efforts. Those who view what happens to them as out of their control are apt to be superstitious and to rely less on past experience. People who are "internals" tend to know more about their own wellness, question health care practitioners more often, and may express less satisfaction at the amount of feedback or information they get about their condition from health care personnel. "Internals" are also more successful in changing the attitudes of others in some situations [2]. In one study, nonsmokers were more internal than smokers [3], and those who quit and did not return to smoking in a specified period of time were more internal than smokers; this last relationship held only for males; females seemed more motivated by others factors such as the tendency to gain weight when not smoking. Internals may choose to go along with or ignore advice when given all the information and alternatives necessary to make a decision; they will, however, resist suggestion if they perceive that they are being manipulated or that others are trying to influence them in subtle ways [4, 5]. Figures 7–1, 7–2, and 7–3 help you to assess the background against which you see your own wellness and the responsibility you are willing to take toward it.

There are numerous studies that support the idea that individuals who have strong beliefs in their ability to control their own destiny are likely to be more alert to information in the environment that provides help for future behavior, take steps to improve the environment, place greater value on skill or achievement rewards and be more concerned with this ability (especially failures), and be resistive to subtle attempts to influence them [6]. Before you read on, it is suggested that you complete the questionnaire found in Figure 7–4. Its format is based on that used by Rotter in his well-known I-E (Internal–External) scale, and the figure may provide useful information for both clients and wellness-enhancers since the score reflects the degree of internality. (See page 316 for a key to scoring.) This kind of assessment can also be helpful by calling attention to the beliefs according to which a person operates. An important question to ask once this assessment has been completed is: Can locus of control be changed? This question is especially relevant for those who are interested in increasing their responsibility for wellness. Some research suggests that locus of control can be changed.

In one study, student counselors changed their locus of control from external to internal once they had become more aware of their muscle activity through electromyographic feedback [7]. This would seem to suggest that if you can learn to tune in to your internal body processes, you are more apt to believe you have control over your fate.

Collar [8] reports that clients become more internal in their locus of control as a result of a specific kind of group counseling called the EPIC model. The EPIC groups followed six exercise units, consisting of perception and feedback skill training; self-disclosure and self-explanation skill building; assessment and understanding of self; personal contracting for change and growth; development of programs for achieving personal growth; and achieving and assessing personal goals and growth. This research suggests that structured exercises that assist clients to focus on themselves and to develop goals and work toward them can increase internality.

Another study looked at the effect of training in success-oriented learning situations for preadolescents [9]. It looked at Rotter's theory that if people receive enough training in success-oriented learning situations to counteract their previous learning, they will begin to attribute successes and failures to their own behavior; in other words, they would become more internal. The results of this study were that externally oriented individuals who were exposed to success at learning tasks became more internally oriented.

Social scientists are developing models for predicting health-related behaviors. The best-developed model for assessing readiness for health teaching is the Health Belief Model [10]. It is used to predict the likelihood that individuals will seek help or change behavior in order to avoid illness. The Model asserts that even when individuals recognize personal susceptibility, they will not take action unless they believe that illness would bring serious physical or social repercussions [11].

People must believe that they could contract the condition before they will engage in preventive health behavior. They also must believe that the condition is serious enough to warrant action. In addition, individuals must believe there are benefits that will accrue from preventive behaviors. For example, people who are convinced that their work environment is unsafe and could lead to cancer may not take action, because they do *not* believe that they can alter their employer's treatment of the environment.

The Model also implies that in order for the necessary wellness behavior to occur, an event must occur (cue to action) that makes individuals aware of their health perceptions and of the need to act [12]. Cues to action could be mass media campaigns, advice from others, reminder postcards or calls from a health care practitioner, the illness of a family member or friend, or a newspaper or magazine article.

General health motivation can also affect health or wellness behavior. People who are concerned about wellness in general are probably more likely to show concern about specific dimensions. Likewise, those who have an ongoing relationship with a health care practitioner are likely to respond favorably when specific advice or teaching is given.

Interventions that arouse fear at a moderate level seem to be the most effective in arousing people to preventive action. In order to elicit action, messages must be accompanied by a specific action recommendation. High fear arousal messages tend to immobilize people or incite massive denial that there is anything to fear [13], at least in situations where individuals are shown a film or asked to read an article. On the other hand, high fear arousal seems beneficial to changing attitudes and behavior when people are more actively involved in the process by taking part in emotional role playing.

Janis reports an experiment where the client plays the role of a person who is suffering from the harmful consequences of cigarette smoking. All clients who took part in the study were smokers; none had expressed interest in cutting down their smoking. Half the group participated in a one-hour role-playing situation, while the other half listened to a tape recording of the role playing. Each client in the role-playing group was asked to pretend he or she was in the physician's office and to behave spontaneously. The experimenter played the role of physician, pointing at an x-ray of the lungs and telling the client that he or she had lung cancer, planning for lung surgery, and asking the other to think over why he or she had not stopped smoking before it was too late. Eighteen months after the role playing, the clients involved in it continued to report a significantly greater decrease in number of cigarettes smoked than those who had listened to the tape. Additional research showed that attitude change increases when clients are given the opportunity to verbalize their own ideas while playing the role [14]. It seems that behavior can be changed toward wellness when clients are taught how to take an active, more responsible role in examining the effects of their harmful behaviors.

Figure 7-5 illustrates the degree to which attitudes to wellness can be affected by the reactions of others. Figure 7-6 gives one way of stopping smoking—an example of responsibility toward one's own health that is so difficult for many to achieve [15]. Figure 7-7 offers a chance to examine your willingness to take responsibility for wellness [16].

HANDLING EMERGENCIES

Part of being responsible is becoming familiar with emergency procedures before emergencies occur.

Samuels and Bennett [17] suggest the first thing to do when confronted with an emergency is to *relax*. Calmness will help people to keep their wits about them, determine the extent of injury quickly, and act in a reasonable way. In addition, approaching the injured person in a calm way will help him or her relax and will help you even if *you* are the injured person. Even in an emergency there is time to close your eyes and take several deep breaths in a slow and rhythmical manner. With each breath, imagine your body relaxing. Once relaxed, it is useful to remind yourself that you will do the best you can do and realize that that is all that can be done.

It often helps to relax the injured person by taking a moment to use the imagining calmness and relaxation methods presented in Chapter 3. The next thing to do is to determine whether the injured person is bleeding, having trouble breathing, or is in shock, and to deal with these problems first. Further information regarding handling emergencies can be gained by referring to entries found in the Appendix.

Sehnert and Eisenberg [18] list some of the most common emergencies as abdominal pain, convulsion, heart attack, poisoning, and shock. Other emergencies presented in this section are choking on food, rape, and bleeding. Figures 7-8 to 7-15 describe methods of handling each emergency [19-33].

CHOOSING A HEALTH CARE PRACTITIONER

It is not an easy task to choose a health care practitioner who meets your needs. If you are reading this book, you will probably want to work with someone who is interested in wellness and holistic health. Wellness requires collaboration, not submission. It may be important to shop around until a comfortable partnership is found. Piper [34] suggests using the following questions as a basis for making this choice:

1. Where did I hear about this person, and what did I hear?
2. What are the person's credentials—skills, training, education, and experience as a healer?
3. What do I know about his or her field of work?

4. Is this person able to work competently with more than one method or else be willing to refer me to other practitioners?
5. Is his or her fee an amount I feel comfortable paying?
6. Is the length of treatment suggested by the practitioner appropriate to the problem?
7. Do I feel comfortable with this person?
8. Does this person explain things to me in language I can understand?
9. Can this person help me keep track of how all my forms of treatment/healing are affecting me?
10. Am I ready to heal this particular disease in my life?
11. Can this person help me to heal?

There are other concerns that may be of interest in choosing a health care practitioner. One is that the person has knowledge about and is willing to share information about self-care without acting as if the body and its care is too mysterious for the owner to know about. Another concern is the practitioner's status as a role model; for example, does the person smoke or allow smoking in the office, or is he or she overweight?

Another concern you may have is that a physician is nutritionally oriented. Since most do not study about nutrition during their medical education, other health care practitioners may be more helpful as consultants in this area. However, it is possible to locate some nutritionally oriented physicians by writing to The International Academy of Preventive Medicine, 10409 Town and Country Way, Suite 100, Houston, Texas 77024.

WHEN AND HOW TO SEEK A HEALTH CARE PRACTITIONER

To many people, their major health care practitioner is a physician. Medical doctors are of most help for the following:

1. assistance in diagnosing and treating illness
2. tests such as x-rays, cultures, blood or urine analysis, to help diagnose diseases such as venereal disease and strep throat, to identify and treat broken bones
3. drugs to help the body heal itself
4. emergencies that clients feel ill-prepared to cope with
5. to obtain immunizations

Plan to come prepared to a health care practitioner so you can ask questions once you are there. Since you may be anxious and/or in pain when visiting a health care practitioner, it is wise to bring along a trusted friend or family member who can ensure that adequate care is received, important questions are asked, and appropriate self-care information is obtained. Figure 7-16 provides some questions it might be appropriate to ask and/or some information to obtain when visiting a health care practitioner. If you are unable to bring a family member or friend, or if you choose to speak for yourself, write down exactly what questions need to be answered and what fears or anxieties are harbored. This list can be read to the health care practitioner to make sure that the points are covered before the visit ends.

It is important to get to know your health care practitioner before you are ill or in need. One way to do this is to make an appointment for the purpose of getting acquainted. Many of the questions that appear in Figure 7-16 can be answered by the receptionist or through your own observations.

Figure 7-17 helps you to assess the way in which you work with your health care practitioner.

Figure 7-18 lists some questions to ask if the physician should suggest surgery [35, 36]. It is recommended that a primary physician be consulted, since even ethical surgeons are often biased toward doing surgery, and that *at least* one other opinion be obtained. (Most Blue Shield plans cover this procedure.) To be effective, a second opinion must be a truly independent opinion. The best way to ensure this is to make sure the second surgeon is aware that only his or her opinion is being sought, and that regardless of the opinion, he or she will *not* do the surgery. This kind of approach removes the financial incentive of surgery and lowers the surgery bias the second surgeon may have.

Some surgical procedures that were once done routinely are now considered outmoded or unnecessary. Surgical procedures currently being questioned because they have been done unnecessarily at times are hysterectomies, tonsilectomies, and removal of the gallbladder and hemorrhoids [37]. It is up to you to be sure you do not receive unnecessary surgery. Blue Shield has a listing of surgical and diagnostic procedures that are ineffective or outmoded. Not only will these procedures not be reimbursed, but you may be subjecting yourself to unnecessary risks by undergoing them. It is your body, and the burden of responsibility lies with you, so be ever-questioning and well-informed regarding these matters. It is best to have a surgeon who is board-certified and who is a member of the American College of Surgeons. Also, it is wise to choose a surgeon who operates several times a week, but not one who is so busy that he or she has no time to answer questions or to tend to your needs [38]. It is probably worth the money and time to telephone a surgeon who has a reputation for doing the procedure when a complex operation is suggested, even if this means a long distance call.

You may also wish to contact the appropriate self-help group (see Appendix). For example, if you are scheduled for a colostomy or ileostomy, you may wish to contact the United Ostomy Association. You might also benefit from reading one or more of the books listed under "Hospitalization and Alternatives."

PEER AND GROUP HELP

There is a tendency for most people to assume that the health care practitioner has *the* answer for their problem. Unfortunately, this view is supported and even promoted by many health care practitioners. Those interested in wellness, on the other hand, strongly promote the idea that people can learn from one another. Perhaps many health care practitioners do not encourage turning to peers for help, because they fear losing control of the relationship and of being the person who wields power through knowledge. Practitioners who use professional terminology surely hope to mystify, rather than collaborate with, their clients, and clearly convey the idea: "I can understand this difficult and complex problem, but you cannot."

It is also true that people frequently give up their autonomy to health care practitioners. They are apt to revere those in the health field and to assume they are not human and do not make mistakes, when in fact health care practitioners are human and do make mistakes. One way to begin to undo this dominant/submissive relationship is to recognize the wisdom each person has. People can make a concerted effort to work together on common problems with their wellness, with particular health care practitioners, or with health care centers or hospitals. They can teach one another parenting and stress reduction and nutritional, assertive-, fitness-, and environment-enhancing skills. They can keep records of their illness/wellness experiences and share these with others. They can agree to meet regularly to share this information—and then ensure the meetings occur and are fruitful. Clients at the same hospital, clinic, or who work with the same group of health care practitioners can also form groups. There is power in numbers, and people who are dissatisfied with health care are more likely to be listened to—and less likely to be branded as complainers—if they form a group and plan strategies to use to make health care more relevant to them. Perhaps one way to begin this effort is for people to meet and talk to others who are waiting for care in waiting rooms in hospitals, clinics, and private practioners' offices.

Some suggestions for forming groups are:

Start a self-help group.

Start a Get to Know Your Body course.

Work to get child-care education in clinics, hospitals, and private practitioners' offices.

Start a local wellness training program for others.

Create a wellness center staffed by trained wellness enhancers.

Start a hot line for problems related to nutrition, stress, parenting, assertiveness, health and hospital care, intimacy/sharing, fitness, or some other aspect of wellness.

Start a parents' group to mobilize around issues related to child health/wellness.

Be an advocate for wellness in your community; support others' wellness attempts.

Lobby to make sure politicians respond to wellness needs.

People can also learn to use one another as resources. Figure 7–19 shows a method small groups can use to solve wellness problems.

YOUR RESPONSIBILITY REGARDING DRUGS YOU TAKE

Many people assume that if a drug is prescribed for them, it is safe to take. This is not necessarily so. Robert J. Temple, a representative of the Federal Drug Administration (FDA) states: "New drugs are always marketed on the basis of comparatively limited information." There is an organized search for expected results, but those not anticipated are not searched for; ". . . other risks, particularly rare adverse effects or those associated with long-term use, usually cannot be documented before marketing . . . so the first few years after marketing are almost invariably a period of new discovery" [39].

If you are taking a newly marketed drug, you may have reactions that have not been anticipated. In other cases, drugs that were thought safe have now been found to be harmful and may have a high risk of death. Darvon is an example of this case; the drug has not been withdrawn from the market despite its high risk, and distribution of patient information sheets regarding its risk are voluntary [40], so you may or may not be made aware of its risks.

Another danger is the continuing manufacture and prescribing of a drug that has been *shown* to be inappropriate. An example of this is the certification of 15 tons of tetracycline in liquid pediatric dosage by the FDA and the finding that 80 percent of the tetracycline prescribed to young children was in the pediatric syrup formulation when this formulation has been *shown ineffective* [41].

Yet another danger is the way information about drugs gets to doctors. Detail men from drug companies are the *single* source of information for physicians during a period when a drug is first prescribed [42]. No doubt this leads to a biased viewpoint on the part of prescribing physicians.

In addition, there are a number of ways in which sources of funding from drug companies to researchers may inappropriately influence the scientific evaluation of drugs. For example, in studies where the principal researcher is not familiar with the design of a study to evaluate a drug, the drug company may assist in a study design that exaggerates the usefulness of a drug and deemphasizes adverse drug effects. Also, when a pharmaceutical firm supports many clinical trials of a drug, a greater therapeutic (good) effect may *seem* to be at work when actually the results may be due to statistical variability [43, 44, 45].

Finally, congressional investigators have found the FDA lax in supervising the testing of new drugs [46]. So, it may be possible that people may be taking prescribed drugs that later turn out to be harmful. You should ask for written information about each drug prescribed for you. It is important to remember that a drug does not have to be proven effective to be prescribed by a doctor or be sold from a drugstore shelf. There are a number of risks involved in taking prescribed or over-the-counter drugs. The first risk is due to the chemical itself and is related to the amount taken. Every drug is a potential poison. For each drug, there is a point at which the harmful effects outweigh the beneficial ones. Prescribers and dispensers euphemistically refer to the harmful effects of drugs as "side effects." In fact, they are not "side effects," but effects of the drug that are known to be harmful. For example, most people consider aspirin to be a rather mild drug, but 10 percent of the adverse drug reactions —such as skin rash, asthma, hives, and bleeding in the digestive system [47]—recorded in hospitals in the United States are due to aspirin. You can locate or purchase a *Physician's Desk Reference* so you can look up any drug that is prescribed, look at the harmful effects of the drug, and discuss this information with the prescribing physician.

The second type of risk is due to allergic reactions to the drug. These are very important because they are unpredictable. The doctor who prescribes a drug cannot know how an individual will react to that drug. Descriptions of drugs found in pharmacology books are the expected reactions, but each person has the capacity to respond in an individualized way.

The third type of risk is that the more drugs are taken, the less effect they may have. For example, certain diuretics (water pills) work at first but lose their effectiveness if taken long term. So do sleeping pills. In the case of antibiotics, "germs" become resistant to these drugs; this has already happened with the bacteria that cause gonorrhea, "staph" infections that are often *acquired in hospitals*, and pneumonia. This problem can be compounded by prescribing anti-biotics for cold symptoms when they are known to be ineffective [48]. If you are given a prescription for a drug such as penicillin when you have a cold, learn to question your physician about this practice.

Some prescribed drugs are so likely to cause drug reactions that their use should be questioned. These drugs are barbiturates, codeine, penicillin, and drugs that are widely prescribed and/or used that are of questionable value—tranquilizers, decongestants, and antihistamines.

This problem is driven home even more clearly when the statistics for drug reactions are examined. Four to seven percent of all hospitalizations are due to adverse drug reactions, and they also account for 30,000 deaths each year [49]. In one study of 714 people followed through their hospital stay, 122 of them had 184 adverse drug reactions. More than 13 percent of the patients suffered a drug-related problem *after* admission to the hospital, and *six* of them *died as a result* [50].

Because of these problems, you need to begin to question the idea that a "magic pill" will result in health or wellness. If you do decide to take prescribed or over-the-counter drugs, be aware that there are dangerous consequences when some drugs interact. For example, combining alcohol and tranquilizers can lead to death, while taking some drugs for depression such as Parnate and then eating cheese or pickled herring or drinking wine or beer can be fatal. Taking MAO inhibitors (a type of drug used to treat depression) and then taking a nasal decongestant, a cough or cold remedy, or an appetite depressant (amphetamine) can trigger a stroke or heart failure in a person who is older or who has high blood pressure. Diuretics are best known for depleting the body of helpful minerals, such as potassium, but when they are combined with digitalis (a heart medication), a serious toxicity problem can result. These are just some of the problems that have to be considered. Potential harm increases geometrically as the number of drugs taken increases.

There may be a 50 to 75 percent chance that each drug prescribed will be taken at the wrong time, in the wrong dosage, or is the wrong drug to be taking. People often think they can change the amount of frequency with which they take the drug. They need to learn to be more concerned about the possible dangers of drugs. You need to become more persistent in asking physicians exactly *what* a drug is for, *when* you should take it, and *why*. Unfortunately, when you buy over-the-counter drugs, you may not have anyone to ask these questions. You may want to take a drug for pain or headache and end up taking a substance that has codeine in it without even knowing it [51].

One way you can increase your responsibility for wellness is to begin to ask the following questions:

1. What drugs am I taking?
2. Do I know the names of them?
3. Do I have a person to ask about the drug or (better yet) do I have a written source, such as the *Physician's Desk Reference* (PDR), that I can refer to for drug information?
4. What is the drug for?
5. What other effects does the drug have besides the one I'm taking the drug for?
6. What potential dangers are there to taking the drug with other drugs?
7. How often should I take the drug for maximum effectiveness?
8. What is the correct amount to take to get the best results?

In many cases you can get some or all of this information from your physician. If he or she does not have the time or inclination to share the information with you, or if you are too flustered or anxious to ask at the time a drug is prescribed, you can telephone your questions or look up the drug in an up-to-date pharmacology book.

In some cases, it is not known what effect one drug will have on another; it is always best to take the least number of drugs possible for this reason. However, there have been studies done on the more common combinations; find a recent book in your library or bookstore that discusses drug interactions.

PROJECTS TO GET INVOLVED IN

There are innumerable projects people can become involved in to begin to take more responsibility for their wellness. Some of these have already been mentioned. Other suggestions appear in Figure 7-20.

Figure 7-1   How Ready Am I to Assume Responsibility for My Own Wellness?

		Yes	No
1.	I believe I am susceptible at this time to something that will decrease my wellness	......	......
2.	This change or condition is apt to have serious physical or social consequences	......	......
3.	I believe this change or condition warrants my swift action to prevent serious consequences	......	......
4.	I believe that if I do act to prevent these consequences, I will reap benefits from doing so	......	......
5.	I have recently become aware of the dangers inherent in not acting to prevent the change or condition	......	......
6.	I have an ongoing relationship with a health care practitioner or a wellness enhancer	......	......
7.	I view myself as a client, not as a passive patient	......	......
8.	I am losing my confidence in health care advice given by scientists, doctors, and/or public officials	......	......
9.	I would welcome information regarding ways I maintain my health and increase my wellness	......	......
10.	I am dissatisfied with the way I feel and/or look, and I am ready to try something new	......	......
11.	I am ready to begin to take charge over what happens to me and my body	......	......
12.	I feel I am at a time in my life when I am open and ready for change	......	......
13.	I will only assume responsibility for wellness if it pleases a health care practitioner and I get approval for it.	......	......
14.	I'll agree to take responsibility for my own wellness in order to avoid being punished by a health practitioner or someone else	......	......
15.	I'll only accept responsibility for my own wellness if an authority figure tells me to	......	......

Figure 7–1 /// 307

	Yes	No

16. I'll accept responsibility for my own wellness if I make a contract with myself or a wellness enhancer to do so   ....

17. I have examined my values and principles and find wellness is in accord with them and is something I want to take responsibility for   ....

Figure 7–2   Choosing Wellness Values

Directions:

A.   Read the statements below and circle the response that most closely indicates the way your parents, friends, industry representatives, or health care practitioners have told you to act.

B.   After circling all responses, go back and for all yeses write an alternative view of how else you might act if someone had not told you how to respond.

1.   a.   My parents always told me to eat everything on my plate.   YES NO

    b.   Alternative view:

2.   a.   My teachers always told me to respect people in authority.   YES NO

    b.   Alternative view:

3.   a.   My health care practitioner always told me not to worry and to just follow his or her advice.   YES NO

    b.   Alternative view:

4.   a.   My parents always told me not to be impolite and push for what I want.   YES NO

    b.   Alternative view:

5.   a.   Commercials and ads tell me highly processed and convenience foods are good for me.   YES NO

    b.   Alternative view:

6.   a.   When I gain weight, my parents tell (told) me, "Don't worry, you look healthy."   YES NO

    b.   Alternative view:

7.   a.   My parents always told me I was sickly and prone to illness.   YES NO

    b.   Alternative view:

Figure 7-2 /// 309

8. a. My parents always taught me to keep my feelings
   to myself and not to share them with others.   YES NO

   b. Alternative view:

9. a. My parents taught me to keep up with the Joneses
   and buy as many possessions and luxury items as
   I could afford.   YES NO

   b. Alternative view:

10. a. My doctor told me not to worry about what my blood
    pressure reading is because he'd look after it.   YES NO

    b. Alternative view:

11. a. When the clock says it's time to eat, I eat, even
    if I'm not hungry or feel upset.   YES NO

    b. Alternative view:

12. a. As long as the government doesn't ban foods or
    products, it's O.K. to use them.   YES NO

    b. Alternative view:

13. a. This country has a pure, fresh water supply,
    and I don't have to worry about drinking what
    comes out of my water tap.   YES NO

    b. Alternative view:

14. a. It's O.K. to have any x-rays as long as they are
    recommended by a physician or dentist.   YES NO

    b. Alternative view:

15. a. People don't like to be touched unless they ask
    to be touched.   YES NO

    b. Alternative view:

16. a. My doctor takes care of my health and makes
    sure I get the right treatment.   YES NO

    b. Alternative view:

(continued)

Figure 7–2 (continued)

---

17. a.   If my doctor orders a test or treatment, I should comply.   YES NO

    b.   Alternative view:

18. a.   My parents taught me not to trust anybody.   YES NO

    b.   Alternative view:

19. a.   My parents taught me to be sure to please other people first, or I won't be liked.   YES NO

    b.   Alternative view:

20. a.   My parents taught me not to think about death, dying, and separations.   YES NO

    b.   Alternative view:

21. a.   I can't change my family or friends, so I may as well do what they want.   YES NO

    b.   Alternative view:

22. a.   It's not my business to know about unsafe practices in my work environment; I get paid to take chances.   YES NO

    b.   Alternative view:

23. a.   If I don't approve of any of the candidates running for office, I just don't vote.   YES NO

    b.   Alternative view:

24. a.   There are all kinds of dangers in the environment, so I might as well not worry about them.   YES NO

    b.   Alternative view:

Figure 7–3 /// 311

Figure 7–3 Taking Charge of My Life

---

1. List any counterproductive beliefs you have that keep you from taking charge of your life; some common ones are: "Other people know better than I do, so I let them take charge of what happens to me"; "I shouldn't take charge of my life, because I don't know how to"; "I shouldn't try to take charge of my life, because it's all a matter of luck or fate anyway." These are only *some* common beliefs or thoughts that prevent people from taking responsibility; list whatever prevents you below, then dispel each counterproductive belief.

Counterproductive beliefs   *Dispelling the belief*

2. Assume you are a unique person with a unique nervous system, brain, body-build, personality, life history, likes/dislikes, resources, and role models. List the ways in which you are unique, and then write a wellness goal for each.

   A. Things unique about my nervous system are:

   One wellness goal I have because of this uniqueness is:

   B. Things unique about my brain and the way I think and act are:

   One wellness goal I have because of this uniqueness is:

   C. Things unique about my body build are:

   One wellness goal I have because of this uniqueness is:

   D. Things unique about my personality are:

   One wellness goal I have because of this uniqueness is:

   E. Things unique about my life history are:

   One wellness goal I have because of this uniqueness is:

(continued)

Figure 7–3 (continued)

F. Things unique about my likes/dislikes are:

One wellness goal I have because of this uniqueness is:

G. Things unique about my resources are:

One wellness goal I have because of this uniqueness is:

H. Things unique about my role models are:

One wellness goal I have because of this uniqueness is:

3. Having a sense of purpose can help you take charge of your life. Begin to develop like goals and strategies for getting there.

A. My aims in life are:

1.

2.

3.

4.

5.

6.

B. I can begin to achieve one of those goals by (list *specific* actions):

1.

2.

3.

4.

Figure 7-3 /// 313

4. Believing you are O.K. and competent to take responsibility for yourself is important. Take a few minutes and jot down several things you feel you are O.K. about.

    A. I am O.K. about

    B. I am O.K. about

    C. I am O.K. about

5. At times you may prefer illness to health, because it offers escape from unpleasant reality, because it brings special attention and care, or because it may mask some inadequacy. Jot down your latest illnesses or physical symptoms, and then take a few minutes to think what these were and what purposes they may have served.

    A. My last illness or physical symptom might have served the purpose of

    B. Other illnesses or symptoms might have served the purpose(s) of

Figure 7–4   Clark Health/Wellness Belief Scale

This questionnaire can be used to find out how different people feel about health and wellness. Each item consists of a pair of alternatives, a and b. Select the statement for each pair with which you most strongly agree or the one you think is true, not the one you think you should choose. There are no right or wrong answers: it is a question of personal belief. Try to respond to each item independently of how you responded to previous items.

Agree

1. a.   I carry the key to my own well-being in the way I choose   .....
         to live   .....

    b.   Health and illness are both matters of luck and beyond
         my control   .....

2. a.   Wellness is a life-long effort   .....

    b.   If I wait, medical science will develop cures for all
         illnesses   .....

3. a.   It matters little whether my health care practitioner
         pursues wellness as long as he/she looks after mine   .....

    b.   I steer clear of health care practitioners who are not
         pursuing their own wellness by not smoking, by
         keeping their weight down, etc.   .....

4. a.   No matter how hard I try, I still get ill (can't stop
         smoking, lose weight, etc.), so I might as well do what
         I want to do   .....

    b.   I have faith in my ability to increase my wellness   .....

5. a.   I have found that if I'm going to be ill, I'm going to
         be ill   .....

    b.   Trusting to fate about my wellness doesn't work; I
         find I have to take a definite course of action   .....

6. a.   Staying well is a matter of hard work, luck has little
         or nothing to do with it   .....

    b.   Staying well is a matter of being in the right place at
         the right time   .....

Figure 7–4 /// 315

			Agree
7.	a.	Environmental pollution has an effect on whether I become ill or not	.....
	b.	Heredity plays a major part in whether I become ill or not	.....
8.	a.	I can have an influence on governmental decisions about wellness	.....
	b.	Politicians, businessmen, and scientific experts make decisions about my wellness	.....
9.	a.	When I devise a wellness plan, I am pretty certain I can make it work	.....
	b.	I don't make long-term wellness plans	.....
10.	a.	Sometimes I feel I have no control over my state of health	.....
	b.	It is impossible for me to believe that my state of health is due to luck or chance all the time	.....
11.	a.	I might as well decide my wellness goals by flipping a coin	.....
	b.	Getting what I want in terms of wellness has little or nothing to do with luck	.....
12.	a.	With enough effort I can begin to decrease the harmful factors in the environment	.....
	b.	It is difficult, if not impossible, to decrease harmful factors in the environment	.....
13.	a.	A good health-insurance plan ought to include incentives for staying well	.....
	b.	A good health-insurance plan should be inexpensive and cover catastrophes like chronic illnesses and heart attacks	.....
14.	a.	It doesn't really matter what I eat, since wellness is unrelated to food	.....
	b.	I should choose what I eat carefully, because it contributes to my wellness	.....

(continued)

Figure 7–4 (continued)

			Agree
15.	a.	I should work at being physically and mentally fit, because both contribute to my wellness and health	.....
	b.	It doesn't matter whether I'm fit or not, since wellness is due to luck and my doctor's prescriptions	.....
16.	a.	Stress is due to factors beyond my control	.....
	b.	I can learn to reduce my stress level and thereby be healthier	.....
17.	a.	If I heal when I'm hurt or ill, it's because something outside me helped me heal, like antiseptic or medicine	.....
	b.	I can learn to use my own healing potential and thereby enhance my wellness	.....
18.	a.	I think it's important to stand up for my rights when I feel others are trampling on them	.....
	b.	It doesn't pay to stand up to others since they don't listen anyway	.....
19.	a.	I question health care practitioners, lawyers, and anyone from whom I purchase a service, because I share the responsibility for what happens to me	.....
	b.	I assume doctors, lawyers, nurses, and other authorities know what I need better than I do	.....
20.	a.	Meeting new friends is a matter of luck	.....
	b.	If I want to meet someone, I should go right up to them and tell them I want to spend more time with them	.....
21.	a.	Pain is something that has to be endured, and it will pass	.....
	b.	When I am in pain, I can take action to reduce my pain	.....

If you agree with the following statements, you are more internal (and apt to take responsibility for your wellness): questions 1a, 2a, 3b, 4b, 5b, 6a, 8a, 9a, 10b, 11b, 12a, 14b, 15a, 16b, 17b, 18a, 19a, 20b, 21b. (Items 7 and 13 are filler items and do not count.)

Copyright 1979 Carolyn Chambers Clark

Figure 7-5 /// 317

Figure 7-5   Controversial Issues Exercise

Directions:

1.   Read the controversial issue statement below.

2.   Do not sign your name, but make one comment illustrating how you feel about the statement or issue (Part A).

3.   Route this paper around to several other people working on wellness issues. Ask each one to read the statement and everyone else's comments without judging them.

4.   When everyone has read each comment, each person is to decide whether he or she feels the same way about the issue now (Part B).

Controversial Issue Statement:
Anyone who wants to smoke should be able to do so whenever and wherever they want.

Part A: My reaction to this statement is:

Part B: Now that I have read others' reactions, I feel the following way about the issue:

Figure 7–6   Ending Smoking

The SmokEnder method seems to be an effective way to help clients stop smoking. The method attempts to change attitudes about quitting. People are asked to describe themselves in detail, including personal appearance, accomplishments, school and work record, social relationships, family relationships, and personal goals. Participants are also asked to look at their feelings of inadequacy and how they act it out through procrastinating or bragging or through trying to impress others or make them feel sorry or hostile toward others. This kind of approach is meant to help smokers to assess who they are and to begin to stop making excuses for themselves or their inadequacies. Jacquelyn Rogers, cofounder of the method, believes that people smoke to decrease anxiety or to reward themselves after a difficult or boring activity [15]. Some of the techniques below might be useful if you wish to quit smoking:

1. Keep a notebook of past and current successes. Look at the list frequently, and remind yourself of your ability to be successful at things you do.

2. Convince yourself you *can* quit; write messages or signs to yourself that you can quit, and concentrate on thinking, "I can quit."

3. Find an intensely personal reason for wanting to quit.

4. Use your list of inadequacies or weaknesses to develop a list of things you can do to improve yourself.

5. Write down all the missed opportunities you regret; choose one that is reachable, and go after it.

6. Make a list of all the things you like to do, and reward yourself with one of them (rather than with a cigarette) each time you feel uncomfortable or bored.

7. Make a list of reasons why you originally started smoking, and compare this list with the reasons for which you now smoke.

8. Decide what you can do to live up to your full potential, and act on it; set one goal for yourself for the coming year.

9. Keep a log of each time you "light up," and categorize each according to its purpose: to get going in the morning or at work or school, in anxious situations, automatically with no apparent reason, to answer the telephone, to promote regularity, to appear calm and collected, to celebrate, to relax, to relieve boredom, to fall asleep, to quell hunger, because it tastes good, to complete a pleasurable cycle (after sex, a good meal, after finishing a project), because certain sounds or smells make you think of a cigarette, to keep your hands busy, to soothe pain or headache.

10. Write a list of things that bug you. Take action to eliminate these things one by one, and draw a dark red line through each as it is eliminated.

Figure 7-6 /// 319

11. If cigarettes are used as a "pick-me-up," substitute six small high-protein meals, sufficient sleep, take a glass of milk or fresh fruit or vegetable juice when feeling fatigued, learn a relaxation exercise, increase your circulation through exercise, and drink a glass of cool or warm water upon arising.

12. End your meals with foods that do not naturally lead to a cigarette; for example, have a glass of milk or a half a grapefruit rather than coffee.

13. Reduce coffee intake—switch to noncaffeinated tea or bouillon.

14. Reach for some pineapple or citrus fruit when feeling "acidy."

15. Drink milk before bedtime (as a way of getting to sleep) and when feeling nervous.

16. Use deep breathing instead of reaching for a cigarette.

17. Realize nicotine is an addictive stimulant and that the nicotine will be out of your system in three or four days.

18. Find someone else who quit smoking who can encourage you and whom you can call *instead* of having a cigarette.

19. Stay away from friends who smoke as much as possible; find new nonsmoking friends.

20. Buy cigarettes by the pack, not by the carton.

21. Buy different brands of cigarettes, and try not to smoke two packs of the same brand in a row.

22. Use the opposite hand from the one you usually use to smoke.

23. Put cigarettes in an unfamiliar place.

24. Develop and maintain a clean mouth taste.

25. Each time you reach for a cigarette, ask, "Do I really want this cigarette?"

26. Develop and prepractice responses to peer pressure comments to smoke, such as: "Come on, one won't hurt you." "Smoking makes you independent, like an adult." "Here, have one."

27. Tell six people, "I've quit smoking, and it was easy."

28. Ask friends, family, and coworkers not to leave cigarettes around or offer you one.

29. When you have an urge for a cigarette, picture the word, "stop" in your mind.

30. Every time you think of having a cigarette, take a deep breath, while pushing your stomach out and clenching your fists; hold your breath briefly, and then exhale and relax.

Figure 7-7 Taking Responsibility for Solving My Problems [18]

Step 1:   Ask yourself the following questions:

Do I really want the answer to my wellness problem?

Do I feel I deserve to be well?

Am I willing to acknowledge the answer to my wellness problem even if it is different from what I hoped for or seems difficult to accomplish?

If the answer to all three questions is "yes," move on to Step 2; otherwise, work on being able to answer a truthful yes to all three. When ready, move on to Step 2.

Step 2:   Use a relaxation technique to relax your body completely.

Step 3:   Close your eyes, and imagine yourself sitting with the three wisest wellness experts in the world. Imagine you ask them to help you solve your wellness problem. Keeping yourself relaxed and centered on this experience, allow yourself to hear whatever answers are forthcoming.

Step 4:   While listening and reflecting on their answers, tell yourself: "I deserve the solution to this problem with my wellness"; feel confident about your ability to solve the problem. Realize that past attempts to solve it were not failures, only delays on the road to success.

Figure 7-8 /// 321

Figure 7-8   Dealing with Abdominal Pain [19, 20]

Step 1:   Assess the situation by asking the following questions and gathering the following information:

When did the pain first appear?

What makes the pain worse (eating, not eating, breathing, physical effort, bowel movement or passage of gas, nervousness)?

Is the pain constant, increasing, or off and on?

Is the pain sharp, dull, burning, cramping, or aching?

Where is pain felt; does the location change?

Is it painful to urinate?

What is the injured person's temperature and pulse? (Retake every 4 hours.)

Is the abdominal area tender or painful to the touch?

Does the abdominal area appear unusual in size, shape, or rigidity?

If the person vomits or feels nauseous, how much, and how often does this occur?

Has the person been near anyone else with similar pain or symptoms recently?

Has the person eaten or drunk an unusual amount or type of food?

Has the person had a recent blow or injury to the stomach area?

Has the person been under a great deal of stress lately?

Step 2:   Keep the person quiet and in a comfortable position.

Step 3:   *Do not* give any of the following: laxatives, enemas, pain medication, heat applications to the abdomen, food, or fluid except ice chips or sips of water.

Step 4:   Call health care practitioner when a pattern of pain has been established and when temperature, pulse, and blood pressure have been recorded.

Figure 7-9   Dealing with Convulsion [21, 22]

Step 1:   Protect the person from being injured on or by surrounding objects.

Step 2:   Roll the person on his or her side to ensure breathing; clear the mouth of vomitus or saliva to making breathing easier.

Step 3:   Keep curiosity seekers away, and time the convulsion.

Step 4:   If person is a stranger, check for evidence (medical or ID tag or card) of epilepsy and medication for it; do this in the presence of a witness to decrease the possibility of being accused of theft. Identify doctor's name from found evidence and call him or her.

Step 5:   If person is a child, take the temperature. If fever goes above 102° rectally (to 103° or 104°), reduce the fever by sponging the child with cool (not cold) cloths or immerse in lukewarm water until fever lowers; then check for injuries, encourage the child to drink fluids after convulsion ends, and then to rest in a cool room.

Step 6:   Call a health professional if any of the following are true:

this is the person's first convulsion

if the convulsion is not accompanied by fever

if a child is under six months' old, or five years old or older, or if the person is an adult

if unable to reduce the temperature to 101°

if the convulsion lasts more than 1 minute

Figure 7-10 /// 323

Figure 7-10   Dealing with Heart Attack [23]

Step 1:   Assess yourself for factors associated with heart attack, including: high cholesterol level, high blood pressure, physical inactivity, cigarette smoking, obesity, and feelings of being continually under time pressures.

Step 2:   If any of the above factors are found, take steps to eliminate them.

Step 3:   Observe for classic signs of heart attack: nausea, clammy skin, difficulty in breathing, pain in chest that radiates into the left arm, and irregular heart beat.

Step 4:   If above signs not evident, check for other signs of heart attack, including:

pain at or above the level of the nipple on both sides of the chest

continuous dull pressure or squeezing sensation under the necktie going up into the neck or jaws

pain associated with sweating

discomfort worse while lying down

distress on the inside of the left arm

pain persists for at least five to ten minutes

Step 5:   If above signs are present, go to the nearest hospital or have someone take you; do not drive. If no one is available, call the rescue squad and ask to be taken to the coronary care unit. Lie down and rest until ambulance arrives.

Figure 7-11   Dealing with Poisoning [24-26]

Step 1:   Lock up medicines if there are children or confused people in your home; throw out medications not currently needed or those that were prescribed and not completely used. Buy medicines with safety caps, if possible. Label all cleaning solvents, gasoline, kerosene, hobby materials, etc., clearly, and keep in a locked or safe place. "Child-proof" your house if children are present. Do not self-medicate.

Step 2:   If poisoning seems probable, try to identify the kind of particular poison taken. Get the bottle or container, and try to estimate how much has been swallowed. Sniff the person's breath; alcohol, kerosene, turpentine, or fingernail polish remover can often be identified in this way. Observe lips, mouth, and skin for evidence of burns from caustic poisons, such as lye. Note for pinpoint pupils; they are a sign of morphine or similar drug poisoning.

Step 3:   If skin has come in contact with poisonous substances, flush the area with large amounts of water; have person stand under a shower or hose them down immediately before removing their clothes. After thorough flushing remove (or ask the person to remove) their clothes.

Step 4:   Give the person a glass of milk to dilute poison without inducing vomiting. If poison can be identified, vomiting can be induced by tickling the back of the person's throat with a finger or by giving a mixture of mustard and water or syrup of ipecac. *DO NOT* induce vomiting when poison is *not* known *or* if poisoning is due to caustic alkalines such as drain cleaner, petroleum products such as gasoline or kerosene, or strong acids such as toilet-bowl cleaner, or if the person is unconscious or having convulsions.

Step 5:   Position the person on his or her side with mouth lower than chest so vomitus is not swallowed.

Step 6:   Call Poison Control Center, report the problem, and ask for advice and help from a rescue squad.

Step 7:   Check and record breathing and pulse rates. Maintain breathing if necessary by removing foreign matter from mouth, tilting head back, pulling jaw down, pinching nostrils closed, placing your mouth on the other's mouth and blowing breath gently into his or her lungs; take your mouth away and listen for exhaled breath. Repeat, breathing 12 times a minute for adults, 20 times a minute for children. Remain with the person until help arrives.

Step 8:   Notify the person's health care professional.

Figure 7-12 /// 325

Figure 7-12   Dealing with Shock [27, 28]

Shock can occur whenever there is an injury or serious emotional shock.

Step 1:   Check for symptoms of shock:

cold, clammy skin;

fast, weak pulse, increasing in rate;

lowering blood pressure;

pale face;

dizziness;

nausea;

dilated pupils.

Step 2:   If symptoms are present:

have the person lie down;

check to be sure there is an open airway and effective breathing; remove vomitus or mucus from his or her mouth;

elevate the legs at least two inches off the ground *unless* there is a chest or head injury;

cover the person with a sheet or blanket(s)—enough to keep him or her warm, but not hot;

give the person small amounts of water, unless there is abdominal injury, unconsciousness, or vomiting;

take and record the pulse every five minutes;

call rescue squad and/or health care practitioner.

Figure 7–13 Dealing with a Choking Emergency:
the Heimlich Maneuver [29, 30]

Step 1:   Stand behind the choking person while wrapping your arms around his or her waist.

Step 2:   Let the person's head, arms, and upper body hang forward.

Step 3:   Make a fist with one hand, grasp it with the other hand and place the fist slightly below the rib cage and slightly above the navel.

Step 4:   Press the fist quickly upward into the choking person's abdomen. Repeat if necessary. If you are choking, press a table or sink just below the diaphragm or use your own fist. If the choking person is lying down, place the person face up and kneel astride his or her hips. Place hands on top of one another with the heel of the bottom hand below the rib cage and above the navel while pressing into the abdomen with a quick upward thrust.

Figure 7–14 /// 327

Figure 7-14   Dealing with Rape [31]

Step 1:   Call a friend or the local crisis hot line or rape crisis center. Ask that person to accompany you to the hospital. Do not change, take a shower, or douche.

Step 2:   Be sure to get a checkup at the hospital; there may be internal injuries you are not aware of.

Step 3:   Be aware that you do *not* have to take estrogen at that time, and that this drug will probably terminate a possible pregnancy but has harmful side effects; remember you can wait until six weeks after your last period and get a pregnancy test and then decide what to do.

Step 4:   Be sure you have a VD test then and *again* in six weeks.

Step 5:   Call the police to report the rape (or have a friend or hospital staff member call for you).

Step 6:   Decide whether or not you want to press charges. You may wish to consult local rape laws and court procedures and talk to others who have been raped as well as to sympathetic lawyers who have had previous experience with rape cases.

Step 7:   If you decide to press charges, improve your chances in court by:

writing down *all* details of the rape experience as soon as possible and sharing them with *your* lawyer only;

making it clear to the police that you want to prosecute;

contacting the police and/or your lawyer to keep up to date on the current status of your case;

calling your lawyer for a pre-trial conference the day before you go to trial;

emphasizing firmly that force was used to make you submit during the rape;

rehearsing your story to be sure you do not contradict yourself;

using anatomical words used by your lawyer only once he or she has used them, so jurors do not equate anatomical knowledge with promiscuity.

Step 8:   Be aware that you will have strong feelings after the trauma of rape, including anger, disgust, humiliation, guilt, horror, and anxiety. Be sure to find at least one other person with whom you can *fully* share these feelings—either a friend or a relative, a crisis counselor, or a counseling group at a rape crisis center.

Figure 7-15   Dealing with Bleeding [32, 33]

Step 1:   Relax and remember that bleeding can almost always be stopped by applying direct pressure to the bleeding area.

Step 2:   Place sterile gauze pads or a clean cloth on the wound, and place your whole hand firmly over the wound; press down hard. If nothing else is available, use your bare hand. Find the place that is bleeding the most, and concentrate your attention there. Maintain pressure for ten minutes without lifting your hand to look at the wound.

Step 3:   If the wound is large, bandage it firmly while continuing to apply pressure. If it is small, evaluate it to see whether stitches are needed. If the cut does not gap out, only the top layer of skin has been cut and the wound will heal by itself. If the cut is minor, wash it out with a great deal of water (several quarts) to get all foreign particles out of it.

Step 4:   If ice is available, apply to the area *around* the wound.

Step 5:   If the bleeding is from an arm, hand, foot, or leg, elevate that part unless there is a broken bone.

Step 6:   If the cut has got dirty material in it, or if it is severe, obtain a tetanus shot from your doctor or health clinic.

Step 7:   Call a health care practitioner if any of the following occur or are needed:

if the wound is large enough to require stitches;

if the person who bleeds is in shock;

if a small cut continues to bleed after applying direct pressure for 20 minutes.

Figure 7–16 /// 329

Figure 7-16   Some Information to Obtain about and from a Health Care Practitioner

---

1. Do you make house calls? If so, what is the fee?

2. What is your fee and what does it include?

3. Who covers for you when you are away?

4. How long a time is allotted for my visit?

5. Do you take telephoned questions?

6. How long can I expect to wait to see you when I have an appointment?

7. Do you mind if I bring a friend or family member with me when I am examined or treated?

8. How do you feel about telling me what you are doing and why as you examine or treat me?

9. Will you give me copies of my laboratory test results?

10. How important do you think vitamins and nutrition are to my health?

11. How do you feel about preventive health care?

12. How will this drug (test, procedure) help me?

     What are the possible good and bad effects? Will you write down specific instructions for me so I'll be sure to get the most benefit from it?

13. What kind of health education or self-care programs do you offer?

14. What can I do to help speed up the healing process?

Figure 7-17 How I Work with Health Care Practitioners

		Yes	No	Some-times
1.	I would welcome information that would help me learn to help myself to higher levels of wellness	......	......	....
2.	I am suspicious of pronouncements about health from government officials and scientists	......	......	....
3.	I resist taking prescribed medications because of their cost	......	......	....
4.	I resist taking prescribed medications because I don't understand what they are for, when to take them, and so on	......	......	....
5.	I "shop around" for doctors until I find one who does what I want	......	......	....
6.	Often, I see a health care practitioner primarily to be reassured that I am O.K., not to prevent illness	......	......	....
7.	I do not go to a health care practitioner often since I view it as a sign of weakness and dependency	......	......	....
8.	When I get depressed, seeing a health care practitioner is the last thing I think about	......	......	....
9.	I am vulnerable to illness and tend to seek out a health care practitioner on a nearly continuous basis	......	......	....
10.	Once I've chosen a health care practitioner, I have complete faith in, and obedience to, whatever is advised	......	......	....
11.	When the health care practitioner answers all my questions and takes time with me, I am more likely to follow his or her advice	......	......	....

Figure 7–17 /// 331

		Yes	No	Some-times
12.	When I visit a health care practitioner, I don't want to ask any questions or hear any answers, all I want to know is what I should do to feel better	......	......	....
13.	I would rather work with the same health care practitioner each time I need help	......	......	......
14.	I don't care whether I see the same health care practitioner as long as he or she is concerned about me when I visit	......	......	....

Figure 7-18 Questions to Ask if Surgery is Suggested [35, 36]

1. What is the diagnosis, and how did you arrive at it?
2. In what percentage of cases does the surgery help?
3. In what percentage of cases does the surgery fail?
4. What is the worst that can happen if I do not have surgery?
5. What alternative treatments could be tried first?
6. What complications are expected as a result of the surgery?
7. What percentage of people get these complications?
8. What is the death rate associated with this operation?
9. What will be removed, repaired, or added to my body during surgery?
10. How long will it take to recuperate from the operation?
11. What anesthesia is planned?
12. Can local anesthesia, self-hypnosis, or acupuncture be used instead of general anesthesia?
13. Who will be administering the anesthesia, and are they qualified*?
14. Where will the operation be done?
15. Could I have outpatient surgery rather than stay in a hospital?
16. Are you board-certified as a surgeon?**
17. Are you a member of the American College of Surgeons?**
18. How many times a week do you operate?

*Try to ensure that either an anesthesiologist or a nurse anesthetist will be administering anesthesia.

**These questions can be answered by reading the diplomas on his or her wall and by consulting the *Directory of Medical Specialists* which is available in community hospital libraries and county medical society offices.

Figure 7–19 /// 333

Figure 7-19   Group Problem Solving*

Time: about 1½ to 2 hours

Group Size: No larger than six people; if group is larger, use a facilitator for every five or six people.

1. The process is explained to participants: one person volunteers to be the client, to state a problem, and to take responsibility for ownership and action related to the problem; the others in the group serve as resources to the client; they give ideas, but they do not judge the client's actions or choices or own the problem.

2. The client states the problem. A facilitator writes it down in the client's own words, encouraging the client to be short and concise. Newsprint is used to write down the problem.

3. The client lists everything that has been tried to solve the problem so far.

4. The resource group and the client brainstorm about how to solve the problem, using one or both of the following phrases: "I wish. . . ." or "How to. . . ." (e.g., "I wish we had a workaholic group" or "How to stop people from overworking").

5. The facilitator concurrently lists the brainstorming ideas.

6. The client chooses three solutions.

7. The client gives the pros and cons of one solution. Objections have to be stated in "how to" terms or "I wish" terms.

8. The client picks the major objection.

9. The resource group analyzes and thinks through with the client how to eliminate the objections; the group asks primarily as a clarifier of the client's thoughts.

10. The resource group looks at the objections and makes suggestions about how to eliminate them without input from the client.

11. The client picks the solution he/she thinks is best and tells how he/she plans to proceed with the solution.

12. The resource group makes other suggestions of where to go with the solution.

*This is based on Gordon's Synectics process.

Figure 7-20   Projects to Get Involved In

Plan a self-study course on some aspect of wellness; become your own authority on you and your wellness.

Take one step toward eating purer food, drinking purer water, and taking in fewer chemicals.

If you or another person received poor health care, protest by writing to key people about your disapproval.

Become familiar with your legislators; let them know about your stand on wellness issues.

Learn about groups that are at high risk for environmental pollution; become active in planning state restrictions for harmful substances.

Find out what highways are being planned in your area; help to plan highways where specific pollutants (carbon monoxide, lead, noise) are least objectionable.

Make sure that hot lunch programs at schools and for the elderly are nutritionally sound and helpful in resisting environmental stressors.

Work to have any industry you are involved with remove hazardous environmental conditions.

Identify schools where asbestos materials have been used; work to have them removed or carefully sealed to prevent deterioration.

Contact the Cooperative League of the USA (1828 L Street, NW, Washington, D.C. 20036) and start a consumer cooperative in housing, food, health, or solar energy.

Join with others in evaluating the wellness content of your local newspaper; work to improve this content.

Write to your senator and representative, and encourage them to back legislation requiring the safety-testing of cosmetics, drugs, and other consumer products that may be pollutants or carcinogens.

Work to make sure consumers have a say in decisions about health care, nutrition, energy, and other wellness issues.

Be informed about governmental regulatory agencies; ensure they do their job.

Boycott industries that have harmful policies.

Actively campaign for zoning and ordinances to decrease noise in local communities.

Police the safety of local water supplies.

Figure 7–20 /// 335

Work to make your local hospital a healthier place.

Enlist the support of your employer to provide employee wellness programs as part of your benefit program.

Get involved in health planning for your area by doing the following: locating and maintaining contact with local Health Systems Agency (HSA) staff people who are sympathetic to consumer involvement; become familiar with the workings of the HSA; make sure there is broad representation on the HSA board; get on the mailing list for all notices and information sent out by the HSA; ensure that public hearings are held in all subareas and are publicized in local newspapers, and that the HSA is responsive to consumers.

Get in touch with public action groups and actively support them with time, energy, and/or money.

Encourage your union to strengthen the Occupational Safety and Health Administration.

Encourage your local radio, television, and newspaper to cover environment-related events.

Pressure voluntary health agencies, such as the American Cancer Society, to develop active preventive programs.

Write letters to the editor of your newspaper, criticizing irresponsible or indifferent officials.

Testify at congressional, state, or local hearings on wellness issues.

Take legal action through medical or drug-related suits if you or a family member has been harmed.

Start a product liability suit if you or any member of your family develops cancer (or other destructive illnesses) following the use of or exposure to a cancer-causing product.

Take action to persuade federal health agencies to change their priorities to preventive and wellness endeavors.

Support health care practitioners who enhance wellness, and boycott those who do not; share this information with family, friends, and others.

Act to obtain all possible information on the carcinogenity and toxicity of chemicals, the newest data on nutrition, stress reduction, and other wellness aspects.

NOTES

1. Julian B. Rotter. "Generalized expectancies for internal versus external control of reinforcement," *Psychological Monographs* 80 (1966), pp. 1-28.
2. E. J. Phares, "Internal-external control as a determinant of amount of social influence exerted," *Journal of Personality and Social Psychology* 2 (1965), pp. 642-647.
3. Bruce C. Straits and Lee Sechrest. "Further support of some findings about the characteristics of smokers and nonsmokers," *Journal of Consulting Psychology* 27, no. 3 (1963), p. 282.
4. William H. James, A. Bond Woodruff, and Warren Werner. "Effect of internal and external control upon changes in smoking behavior," *Journal of Consulting Psychology* 29, no. 2 (1965), pp. 184-186.
5. Julian B. Rotter, "Generalized expectancies," p. 24.
6. Ibid., p. 25.
7. Vincent N. Scalese. "Effects of electromyographic feedback training on the perception of locus of control and accuracy of person perception of externally controlled therapist trainees." Unpublished doctoral dissertation, Western Michigan University, 1978.
8. Charles F. Collar. "The effective personal integration model and its impact upon locus of control with clients in group counseling." Unpublished doctoral dissertation, North Texas State University, 1977.
9. Paul James Companik. "Assessment of the attempts to modify locus of control orientation in preadolescent school children." Unpublished doctoral dissertation, The University of Wisconsin—Madison, 1977.
10. *Proceedings of the National Heart and Lung Institute Working Conference on Health Behavior.* Ed. by Stephen M. Weiss. Bethesda, Md.: Department of Health, Education and Welfare, 1975, pp. 42-45.
11. Marshall H. Becker. "The health belief model and sick role behavior," *Health Education Monographs* 2, no. 4 (1974), pp. 409-419.
12. Stephen M. Weiss (ed.). *Proceedings of The National Heart and Lung Institute Working Conference On Health Behavior.* DHEW Publication No. (NIH) 76-868, Bethesda, Md.: National Institutes of Health, 1975, pp. 42-43.
13. Ibid., pp. 43-44.
14. Irving L. Janis (ed.). *Personality: Dynamics, Development, and Assessment.* New York: Harcourt, Brace and World, 1969, pp. 141-144.
15. Jacquelyn Rogers. *You Can Stop.* New York: Pocket Books, 1977, p. 14.
16. Anne Kent Rush. *Getting Clear.* New York/Berkeley: Random House/Bookworks, 1973.
17. Mike Samuels and Hal Bennett. *The Well Body Book.* New York: Random House, 1973, p. 286.
18. Keith W. Sehnert and Howard Eisenberg. *How to Be Your Own Doctor (Sometimes).* New York: Grosset and Dunlap, 1975, p. 64.
19. Sehnert and Eisenberg, *Be Your Own Doctor*, pp. G59-G62.

20. Toni M. Roberts, Kathleen McIntosh Tinker, and Donald W. Kemper. *Healthwise Handbook*. Garden City, N.Y.: Doubleday, 1979, pp. 24-27.
21. Sehnert and Eisenberg, *Be Your Own Doctor*, pp. G62-G63.
22. Roberts et al. *Healthwise Handbook*, pp. 81-82.
23. Sehnert and Eisenberg, *Be Your Own Doctor*, pp. G64-G66.
24. Ibid., pp. G68-G70.
25. Roberts et al., *Healthwise Handbook*, pp. 157-158.
26. Samuels and Bennett, *Well Body Book*, p. 293.
27. Sehnert and Eisenberg, *Be Your Own Doctor*, pp. G72-G73.
28. Roberts et al., *Healthwise Handbook*, pp. 159-160.
29. Sehnert and Eisenberg, *Be Your Own Doctor*, pp. 307-310.
30. "How to handle a choking emergency," *Prevention* (June 1975), pp. 79-81.
31. Boston Women's Health Book Collective. *Our Bodies, Ourselves*, 2nd ed. New York: Simon and Schuster, 1976, pp. 158-161.
32. Roberts et al., *Healthwise Handbook*, pp. 145-146.
33. Samuels and Bennett, *The Well Body Book*, pp. 287-289.
34. Lorin Piper. "Choosing a holistic practitioner." In *The Holistic Health Handbook*, compiled by the Berkeley Holistic Health Center. Berkeley, Calif.: And/Or Press, 1978, pp. 116-117.
35. "How to avoid operations you don't need," *Woman's Day* (April 24, 1979), pp. 12, 128-132.
36. Robert S. Mendelsohn. *Confessions of a Medical Heretic.* Chicago, Ill.: Contemporary Books, 1979, pp. 63-64.
37. Subcommittee on Oversight and Investigations of the Committee on Interstate and Foreign Commerce, House of Representatives. *Cost and Quality of Health Care: Unnecessary Surgery.* Washington, D.C.: U.S. Govt. Printing Office, January, 1976.
38. "How to avoid operations you don't need."
39. Robert S. Temple et al. "Adverse effects of newly marketed drugs," *New England Journal of Medicine* 300, no. 18 (1979), pp. 1046-1047.
40. "New warning on propoxyphene" (Darvon), *FDA Drug Bulletin* 9, no. 4 (1979), p. 22.
41. Wayne A. Ray, Charles F. Federspiel, and William Schaffner. "The malprescribing of liquid tetracycline preparations," *American Journal of Public Health* 67, no. 8 (1977), pp. 762-763.
42. R. R. Miller. "Prescribing habits of physicians: a review of studies on prescribing drugs," *Drug Intell. Clin. Pharmacy* 8 (1974), pp. 81-91.
43. Edward L. Petsonk. "Conflicts of interest in drug research," *New England Journal of Medicine* 301, no. 6 (1979), p. 335.
44. Alfred O. Berg. "Some non-random views of statistical significance," *The Journal of Family Practice* 8, no. 5 (1979), pp. 1011-1014.
45. John Prutting. "Should an antidepressant be combined with a tranquilizer," *New England Journal of Medicine* 300, no. 7 (1979), p. 372.
46. "FDA accused of laxity," *New York Times*, July 25, 1976.
47. "Aspiring: good news, bad news," *Saturday Review* (November 25, 1972), pp. 60-62.

48. Donald M. Vickery. *Life Plan for Your Health.* Reading, Mass.: Addison-Wesley, 1978, pp. 37–39.
49. Edward Kennedy. "Report as Chairman of the Senate Health Committee," *Journal of the American Pharmaceutical Association* (October 1973).
50. Vickery, *Life Plan.*
51. "A case in point: tylenol #3," *Prevention* (December 1976), p. 98.

appendix

Wellness Resources

ASSERTIVENESS

Assertive Skills for Nurses by Carolyn Chambers Clark (Wakefield, Mass.: Nursing Resources, 1978). A workbook based on the module approach to learning. Pre- and posttests are available for each module (differentiating assertiveness from avoiding and aggressive behavior; what hinders and necessitates assertiveness in nursing; assertive assessments; assertive procedures and strategies; work orientation and habits; giving/taking criticism/ help; control of anxiety, fear, and anger). Designed for individual or group self-study or for use as a focus for a workshop or course.

Don't Say YES When You Want to Say NO by Herbert Fensterheim and Jean Baer (New York: Dell, 1975). Uses a behavior therapy approach. Strong in the following areas: achieving a social network, having a close relationship, changing habits, decreasing depression, getting thin, and assertion on the job.

How to Become an Assertive Woman by Bryna Taubman (New York: Pocket Books, 1976). This very readable book presents assertiveness from the viewpoint of both the woman who works outside the home and the woman who works at home. A very common-sense approach to assessing your assertiveness; also, some help with ways of becoming more assertive.

The Mouse, the Monster and Me by Pat Palmer (San Luis Obispo, Calif.: Impact, 1978). A book dedicated "to children who wish to be free and to adults who will help them." This book tackles the issues of assertiveness for children and of children's rights. Available from the publishers, P.O. Box 1094, San Luis Obispo, Calif. 93406.

` *Special Techniques in Assertiveness Training for Women in the Health Profession* by Melodie Chenevert (St. Louis: C. V. Mosby, 1978). A highly humorous and entertaining approach to assertiveness. Based on Transactional Analysis (parent tapes, child tapes, adult tapes, with assertiveness being the use of adult-to-adult communication.)

When I Say No, I Feel Guilty by Manual J. Smith (New York: Bantam, 1975). This book is especially strong in the use of persistence techniques in assertiveness such as Broken Record, Fogging, Negative Assertion, and Negative Inquiry.

CANCER

Cancer Information Service, funded by The National Cancer Institute, HEW, provides information about all aspects of cancer to the general public and to clients who have cancer, as well as to their families. Confidential. Call: 800-555-1212 to obtain the number of the local Cancer Information Service or call The National Office at 800-638-6694.

The Candlelighters, a self-help group of parents of young cancer patients. Seeks to obtain consistent, adequate federal support for research and to help parents who share this difficult experience. There are 65 groups in 38 states, in England and in Canada. Write: The Candlelighters, 123 C. St., S.E., Washington, D.C. 20003 or call 202-544-1696.

CANPATANON (Cancer Patients Anonymous), a self-help peer group that meets regularly to share information, experiences, and hope so that it may cope with the problems confronting a person with a life-threatening illness. Write: Cancer Patients Anonymous, 1722 Ralph Ave., Brooklyn, N.Y. 11236 or call 212-649-3481.

Getting Well Again by Carl O. Simonton, M.D., and Stephanie Matthews-Simonton, R.N. (New York: J. P. Tarcher, 1978). A self-help guide to overcoming cancer for clients and their families.

The Politics of Cancer by Samuel S. Epstein (San Francisco, Calif.: Sierra Club Books, 1978). A very well-written and researched book. Provides invaluable information on environmental sources of cancer, on governmental lack of focus on cancer prevention, and on ineffective prevention of the release of hazardous substances into the environment, including industry opposition to the implementation of laws and regulations and unresponsive governmental agencies who have often been subverted from their missions by political pressures. Dr. Epstein, a physician and professor of occupational and environmental medicine at the School of Public Health, University of Illinois, urges public recognition that most cancer is preventable through concerted action on the political and personal level.

You Can Fight for Your Life—Emotional Factors in the Causation of Cancer by Lawrence LeShan (New York: M. Evans, 1977). This book is useful to those who have cancer, those who wish *not* to develop cancer, for family and friends of those who do develop cancer, and for wellness enhancers. Lawrence LeShan has worked as a psychotherapist with numerous clients who have cancer; he has found a similar core of lack of interest or hope for the future, unresolved loss, and undeveloped self. He gives suggestions for enhancing wellness in clients who have been labeled, "terminal."

CRISIS

Against Rape by Kathleen Thompson and Andra Madea (New York: Farrar, Straus and Giroux, 1974). A comprehensive book (written by two women involved in a rape crisis center) that covers all aspects of the prevention and treatment of rape.

Learning to Say Goodbye: When a Parent Dies by Eda LeShan (New York: Macmillan, 1976). This is an extremely useful book for children and surviving spouses. It can be the focus for preventing guilt and undue resentment in children who lose a parent through death.

Rape: Victims of Crisis by Ann Wolbert Burgess and Linda Lytle Holmstrom (Bowie, Md.: Robert J. Brady, 1974). Provides a good discussion of women's reactions to rape and to the attitudes of the police, courts, health care personnel, family, and friends. It also describes an innovative Victim Counseling Program at Boston City Hospital and is useful to those counseling rape victims. For $6.95 (paper).

EDUCATIONAL MATERIALS

The Consumer Information Catalog: A Catalog of Selected Federal Publications of Consumer Interest developed by The Consumer Information Center, Pueblo, Colorado 81009. Mostly free or minimal-cost publications on subjects such as: child care, consumer protection, diet and nutrition, health, diseases and common ailments, medicine and drugs, home energy conservation.

Decisions about Drinking, prepared by Caspar Alcohol Education Program. Each package contains a Teacher's Guide, Resource Materials, and individualized unique teaching plans for a program spanning from five to ten class periods at each grade level. The material covers alcohol facts, attitudes, decision-making, and alcoholism and is reproducible for convenient classroom use. The series was revised in 1978. Order from: CASPAR Alcohol Education Program, 226 Highland Avenue, Somerville, Mass. 02143.

HealthRight, published by Women's Health Forum. HealthRight, Inc. is a nonprofit women's health education and consumer advocacy organization that researches and publishes pamphlets on women's health concerns, publishes a quarterly newsletter, runs a client advocacy program, and conducts Know Your Body courses. Contact: HealthRight, Women's Health Forum, 175 Fifth Avenue, New York, N.Y. 10010, 212-674-3660.

The Learning Exchange, a consumer-bartering telephone referral service that acts as a clearinghouse, matching people who want to learn with those who want to teach. Has a catalog of more than 3,000 subjects. Write: The Learning Exchange, P.O. Box 920, Evanston, Ill. 60204 or call 314-273-3383.

National Clearinghouse for Alcohol Information (NCALI) provides general information, announcements, and pamphlets on alcohol abuse and alcoholism as well as posters, films, and research abstracts. Write: NCALI, P.O. Box 2345, Rockville, Md. 20852.

The National Women's Health Network publishes the *Network News* bimonthly; it includes the latest women's health information, health feature articles, information on current health policy decisions, articles on local issues relevant to women's health, a conference calendar, and a health hot line. The organization monitors the activities of federal agencies such as the Department of Health, Education and Welfare, including the Food and Drug Administration and the National Institutes of Health, it keeps abreast of Congressional hearings and testimony, and it provides a national resource file on selected women's health issues through the Women's Health Clearinghouse. The Clearinghouse will gather and process information on particular health topics for members. For information, write: National Women's Health Network, 1302 18th Street, N.W., Suite 203, Washington, D.C. 20036.

Plays for Living by the Family Service Association of America. These are professionally written plays that deal with everything from retirement to teenage sex. The plays are half-hour dramatizations of contemporary issues, which attempt to focus community attention on situations that need understanding, discussion, recognition, and action. Most plays end with a question to stimulate discussion. In many places, performances are given by professional actors; in others, amateur and college groups perform. For further information write: Plays for Living, Family Service Association of America, 44 E. 23rd Street, New York, N.Y. 10010.

The School Health Curriculum Project, a primary grade curriculum developed under contract between HEW's Center for Disease Control and The American Lung Association in cooperation with the Seattle School District No. 1. The Project requires that a school entering it sends a full team for training, including two classroom teachers for the grade level for which the training unit is being offered, the principal, and one or two other school personnel, such as school nurse, health educator, curriculum specialist, librarian, or audiovisual coordinator. Workshops are offered throughout the country, primarily in the summer. The curriculum teaches children how their bodies function, what affects their bodies, and how to make good health choices throughout their lives. Write: U.S. Department of Health, Education, and Welfare, Public Health Service, Center for Disease Control, Bureau of Health Education, Atlanta, Georgia 30333.

The YMCA Family Communication Skills Center is a national program offering basic programs (Positive Parenting, Positive Partners, Peoplemaking Thru Family Communication, Valuing Families, Family Enrichment Program, and Family Under-Stand-In) for families. The workshops offer skill training in basic communication. The Skills Center assists in obtaining professional leaders and materials to sponsor workshops in local communities. For additional information write: National YMCA Family Communication Skills Center, 350 Sharon Park Drive, A-23, Menlo Park, Calif. 94025.

ENVIRONMENT

Citizen Action Packet on Emergency Response Planning for Nuclear Accidents, a citizen's handbook explaining what individuals can do to prepare their localities and state governments for radiological accidents. Available from Critical Mass Energy Project, P.O. Box, 1538, Washington, D.C. 20013. Cost: $4.75.

Citizen Action Packet on the Transportation of Radioactive Materials, includes model legislation and background material on the risks posed by the transportation of radioactive materials over our highways, rails, and through our airports. Available from Critical Mass Energy Project, P.O. Box 1538, Washington, D.C. 20013. Cost: $1.00.

HEALTH CARE DELIVERY

Confessions of a Medical Heretic by Robert S. Meldelsohn, a physician who exposes the dangers of hospitals, medications, and doctors. Raises some pertinent issues regarding the disadvantages of the medical model. Provides suggestions for dealing with doctors and educating them so they will be more able to work as preventive health practitioners. Available from Contemporary Publishers, Chicago, Ill., 1979.

Witches, Midwives, and Nurses—A History of Women Healers by Barbara Ehrenreich and Deirdre English (Old Westbury, N.Y.: The Feminist Press, 1973). Explains the rise of male medical professionals and the suppression of women healers since the 14th century. Available from the publisher, P.O. Box 334, Old Westbury, N.Y. 11568, $1.25 (paper).

Worry Clinics sponsored by local Mental Health Associations. The clinics revolve around basic themes: marital problems, middle-age, finances, problems of the working wife, and child-rearing. For additional information, contact: National Association for Mental Health, 1800 Kent Street, Rosslyn, Arlington, Virginia 22209.

HOSPITALIZATION AND ALTERNATIVES

Children in Hospitals, a nonprofit organization comprised of professionals and parents formed to educate all concerned with the needs of children and parents during hospitalization. They publish a list of recommended books and articles and furnish questions parents need to ask regarding hospitals before admitting their children. Write to: Children in Hospitals, 31 Wilshire Park, Needham, Mass. 02192.

Living with Surgery, before and after by Paul J. Melluzzo, M.D. and Eleanor Nealon (Dayton, Ohio: Lorenz Press, 1979). This book deals with mastectomy, colostomy, ileostomy, amputation, hysterectomy, neurosurgery, kidney transplantation, surgery for birth defects, and open-heart surgery. It covers in detail pre- and postoperative procedures and the physical aspects of each operation. It addresses physical and emotional aspects. Recommended for those who are faced with surgery and their families.

The People's Hospital Book written by two doctors, Ronald Gots and Arthur Kaufman (Avenel, N.J.: Crown Publishers, 1978). Offers down-to-earth suggestions, including ten questions to ask your doctor during your hospital stay, one precaution to take before accepting any medication, measures to take to make hospitalization easier for children, suggestions for easing post-surgery discomfort, how to complain effectively about care, ways of ensuring the safety and comfort of an elderly or incapacitated friend or relative, and how to prepare for surgery. Available from the publishers, Dept. 785, 34 Engelhard Ave., Avenel, N.J. 07001.

Physician's Desk Reference (Oradell, N.J.: Medical Economics Company). Yearly supplements are available. This manual provides information on drugs in use including when it is used, when it should not be used, warnings and precautions when using the drug, adverse reactions to expect, recommended amounts to take, and directions for use.

Post-Mastectomy—A Personal Guide to Physical and Emotional Recovery by Win Ann Winkler (New York: Hawthorne Books, 1976). This book is written by a woman who had a modified radical mastectomy. The book deals with the decision to have a mastectomy, the operation, initial fears, first steps in the hospital, and what to expect in subsequent months. Diet, physical activity/exercise, beauty care, health, and postmastectomy clothing are all discussed.

Visiting Nurses' Association is available in most communities to give skilled nursing care at home. Look in yellow pages under nurses.

NUTRITION

Blind Dates: How to Break the Codes on the Foods You Buy. Developed by the Consumer Protection Board of The State of New York. Write: State Consumer Protection Board, 99 Washington Avenue, Albany, N.Y. 12210.

Confessions of a Sneaky Organic Cook, or How to Make Your Family Healthy When They're Not Looking. Written by Jane Kinderlehrer (Bergenfield, N.J.: The New American Library, 1971). Contains easy-to-read information about healthy eating, vitamins, minerals, how to begin to enhance wellness in eating patterns, and delicious recipes. A Signet book available from the publisher, P.O. Box 99, Bergenfield, N.J. 07621.

A Consumer's Guide to Food Additives. Developed by The City of New York's Consumer Affairs Department. Covering a wide variety of subjects, including ways consumers can take action against additives. Available for 35¢ from 80 Lafayette Street, New York, N.Y. 10013.

Diet for a Small Planet, revised edition, by Frances Moore Lappe (New York: Ballantine, 1975). This book is a wealth of information on protein: how to calculate each person's need for it; how to prepare economical low-calorie complete protein meals without meat; why it is important to eat low on the food chain; protein myths; the body useability of various sources of protein, and much more.

Feed Your Kids Right, Dr. Smith's Program For Your Child's Total Health by Lendon Smith (New York: McGraw-Hill, 1979). A pediatrician provides a nutritional program to help prevent many physical illnesses and behavior problems in children. He explains why there is a widespread need for food supplements, and provides data to back up the relationship between hyperactivity and carbohydrate metabolism, acne and zinc, skin rashes and Vitamin A, bedwetting and magnesium, respiratory infections and Vitamin C, and much more.

The Feingold Cookbook for Hyperactive Children and Others with Problems Associated with Food Additives and Salicylates by Ben and Helene Feingold (New York: Random House, 1979). This book shows parents how to prepare dishes that contain no harmful chemicals. It also gives advice on the following: facts on other childhood disorders that may respond to the Feingold diet, a list of foods that contain salicylates, information on other food additives on the market, a method for determining children's sensitivity to foods, advice on other foods that may cause problems, the best sources of Vitamin C for hyperactive children, tips on vitamin supplements, and special precautions about pediatric medications.

Nutrition, Health, and Activity Profile developed by the Wholistic Health and Nutrition Institute. This is a four-page computerized questionnaire designed to teach nutritional basics while emphasizing other wellness dimensions. For more information, write to: N.E.W.S. c/o James M. Cloud, Building C, 150 Shoreline Highway, Mill Valley, Calif. 94941.

Safe Food Guide by Barbara LeDuc (Ringwood, N.J.: J. P. Mauld, Inc., 1976). Lists over 3,000 food items that are free of artificial coloring and flavoring.

PARENTING

How to Father by Fitzhugh Dodson (New York: New American Library, 1974). This book discusses the developmental stages of children from birth to school age, with emphasis on the father's role. There are good appendices on games, books, toys, and readings for parents.

P.E.T. Parent Effectiveness Training by Thomas Gordon (New York: Plume, 1975). This book can be used in self-study by parents who wish to improve their parenting skills by enhancing their communication with their child. Parents can take an eight-week course based on P.E.T. or become an authorized P.E.T. instructor by writing to: Dr. Thomas Gordon, Effectiveness Training Associates, Inc., 110 S. Euclid Ave., Pasadena, Calif. 91101.

Systematic Parent Training by William Miller (Champagne, Ill.: Research Press, 1975). This book describes behavioral modification principles and their application to parenting.

PREGNANCY AND ADOPTION

The Adoption Advisor by Joan MacNamera (New York: Hawthorne Books, 1975). This book is a complete resource for people who are considering adopting a child.

Infertility: A Guide for the Childless Couple by Barbara Eck Menning (Englewood Cliffs, N.J.: Prentice Hall, 1977). This book deals with both the physical and psychological sides of infertility and offers suggestions about where to go for advice and tests and how to proceed regarding the causes and cures.

The International Childbirth Education Association publishes The Pregnant Patient's Bill of Rights and Responsibilities. Complimentary copy sent in return for a stamped, self-addressed envelope. Write ICEA Publication/Distribution Center, P.O. Box 9316, Midtown Plaza, Rochester, N.Y. 14604.

Pregnancy after 35 by Carole Spearin McCauley (New York: E. P. Dutton, 1976). This book describes in detail the risks of late pregnancies. Myths are dispelled; women in their mid-thirties and even forties have an excellent chance of giving birth to healthy babies if the mother has a history of good nutrition and health as well as early and thorough prenatal care.

RESPONSIBILITY

ACLU (American Civil Liberties Union) can refer clients to a lawyer and inform them of their rights. 212-725-1222.

A Citizen's Handbook on Solar Energy. A layperson's introduction to solar power, including consumer tips for buying solar equipment and ideas for citizen action. Available from Public Interest Research Group, P.O. Box 19312, Washington, D.C. 20036. Price $3.50.

Consumer Product Safety Commission is a federal agency that receives reports on injuries/deaths related to hazardous products and assists consumers in evaluating the safety of products on sale to the public. Call: 800-638-2666 (Continental U.S.) or 800-492-2937 (Maryland).

Environmental Defense Fund, Inc., founded for protection of public interest in environmental quality, energy, health and consumer welfare, through legal action based on scientific evidence combined with legal work. Write: Environmental Defense Fund, 475 Park Ave., South, New York, N.Y. 10016 or call 212-686-4191.

Information Packet on Radioactive Waste, includes question-and-answer sheet about radioactive waste and background on waste problems. Summarizes the Government Accounting Office findings and highlights problems involved in the underground disposal of high-level waste. Available from Critical Mass Energy Project, P.O. Box 1538, Washington, D.C. 20013. Cost: $1.00.

National Solar Heating and Cooling Information Center, funded by HUD and the Department of Energy. Provides information concerning the availability of solar heating and cooling installations. Call: 800-523-2929 (U.S.) or 800-462-4983 (Pennsylvania).

Occupational Safety and Health Administration (OSHA) is a federal agency that provides information to workers and accepts reports about health-related accidents or dangerous working conditions. Call: 800-555-1212 for regional OSHA toll-free numbers.

Sierra Club, a citizen's organization founded to make the public more aware of ecological, environmental, and natural resources crises facing the world.

Citizen Energy Project offers a publication list dealing with advocacy and organizing efforts regarding nuclear and solar energy. Write: Citizen Energy Project, 1413 K St., N.W., 8th Floor, Washington, D.C. 20005.

A Consumer's Guide to Taking over Health Planning developed by Ralph Nader's Public Citizen Health Research Group (2,000 P. St., N.W., Washington, D.C. 20036). Suggestions for how to participate in your community's health planning (HSA). $2.00.

Getting Yours: A Consumer's Guide to Obtaining Your Medical Record. A handbook that tells how to assert your right of access to your medical records and why this is important. Available from Public Citizen Publications, P.O. Box 19404, Washington, D.C. 20036. Price $2.30.

Interagency Council on Smoking and Health has developed a Non-Smokers' Bill of Rights. Write: Interagency Council on Smoking and Health, 419 Park Avenue, South, Room 1301, New York, N.Y. 10016.

Organizing for Health Care: A Tool for Change 1974 by the Source Collective, Beacon Press, Boston, Mass. This is a directory of facilities and programs that maximize self-sufficiency and self-protection.

People's Lobby provides information for citizens about how they can use the initiative and referendum on both the state and national levels. Write: People's Lobby, 3456 W. Olympic Blvd., Los Angeles, Calif. 90019.

Public Citizen Congressional Voting Index. A booklet that tells how your Senators and Representatives voted on 40 key consumer, environmental, tax, and government subsidy issues in 1978. Available from Public Citizen Publications, P.O. Box 19404, Washington, D.C. 20036. Price $2.00.

Public Citizen's Health Research Group, founded by Ralph Nader, to present the consumer, client, and worker point of view in matters of health, safety, and health research. Helps public citizen groups organize to work for stated aims and goals. Write: Public Citizen's Health Research Group, 2000 P. St., N.W., Washington, D.C. 20036 or call 202-293-9142.

Through the Mental Health Maze, A Consumer's Guide to Finding a Psychotherapist, Including a Sample Consumer/Therapist Contract by Sallie Adams and Michael Orgel (Washington, D.C.: Health Research Group, 1975). This book provides a wealth of information for clients contemplating psychotherapy, including what to do in case of a mental health "emergency," the client's responsibilities regarding seeking out and working with a psychotherapist, a sample client-therapist contract, elements to consider when drawing up a contract, what to expect from a relationship with a good therapist, common medication used in treatment, definitions of types of therapy, and tests used in psychological evaluation. For a copy write the publisher, 2000 P Street, N.W., Washington, D.C. 20036, 202-872-0320.

SELF-CARE

Exercise and Weight Control. A brochure describing the value of exercise in maintaining proper weight and energy expenditures for 34 activities. Developed by the President's Council on Physical Fitness and Sports and available from the Superintendent of Documents, U.S. Gov't. Printing Office, Washington, D.C. 20402.

Getting Clear, Body Work for Women by Anne Kent Rush (New York:

Random House/Bookworks, 1973). This book is written in a highly readable style and is well illustrated. It can help women become more attuned to their bodies and learn to like themselves. Some of the topics covered are: body awareness exercises; reclaiming your genitals; centering, breathing, and belly power; talking to yourself; language, size, and self-image; relating to your doctor; pain; food awareness; pelvic self-examination; how to choose a therapist; reclaiming your sexuality; massage; anger and sex; couples and communication; long-term relationships: intimacy and sex; menstruation; abortion; pregnancy and childbirth; the child in you: play therapy; deep fantasy; meditation; healing; getting older; and dying.

The Harvard Medical School Health Letter published by Harvard University. A monthly report geared toward preventive medicine and toward helping readers to take care of their health, judge medical information, and learn about the latest developments in medicine. For a subscription, write: Harvard University Press Building, Dept. NYBA, 79 Garden Street, Cambridge, Mass. 02138.

Health Activation Black Bag Learning Series, developed by The Health Activation Network. The series consists of six interactive learning sessions in self-care and has an overriding theme of body observation, including Talk of Your Body, Stethoscope Probes, Body Cavity Investigation, Common Illnesses, The Body Responds to Change, Oral Health, and Nutritional Assessment. Write: P.O. Box 923, Vienna, Virginia 22180, 703-938-4447.

Health Activation for Senior Citizens, developed by Health Activation Network. A guide to assist you to plan, develop, and implement a course that includes sessions on responsibility; the medicine chest; choosing and utilizing health professionals; listening to your body; self-help for medical skills and vital signs, medical emergencies, common conditions, and common injuries; oral-dental health, foot health, yoga, nutrition, alcoholism, and medicine; response-ability to live. Write: P.O. Box 923, Vienna, Virginia 22180.

The Healthscription: A Self-Guide to Wellness by James M. Cloud (Mill Valley, Calif.: W.H.N. Institute, 1977). A workbook containing self-assessment profiles and guides to personal health responsibility. Assists clients in developing a personal approach to stress management, nutrition, physical fitness, and self-responsibility for well-being. Available from W.H.N. Institute, 150 Shoreline Highway, Mill Valley, Calif. 94941. $10.00.

Healthwise Handbook by Toni M. Roberts, Kathleen McIntosh Tinker, and Donald W. Kemper (Garden City, N.Y.: Doubleday, 1979). This book is devoted to measures to take to prevent, recognize, and treat common illnesses. It was developed through Healthwise, Inc., a nonprofit organization committed to encouraging self-care of routine health problems.

How to Be Your Own Doctor (Sometimes) by Keith W. Sehnert, with Howard Eisenberg (New York: Grosset and Dunlap, 1975). Offers information regarding decisions about when you need to see a physician and when you can simply and safely handle the problem yourself. The Self-Help Medical Guide, pp. G-1–G-128 are the most useful.

Medical Self-Care. A journal dedicated to people taking responsibility for their own health. Write to: Tom Ferguson, Editor, Box 31549, San Francisco, Calif. 94131. Write to same address for workshops on self-care in your area.

The Mind/Body Effect by Herbert Benson (New York: Simon and Schuster, 1979). This book is in the spirit of wellness. Dr. Benson is the author of *The Relaxation Response*, and an Associate Professor of Medicine at Harvard Medical School. In this new book, he shows how clients are largely responsible for their own health, that they are generally well when *they* feel well, how the risks of modern medicine can be minimized, and how clients have a *right* to be well for as long as possible. Some topics discussed are: Why hope is the best medicine; why high blood pressure can be a reaction to preoccupation with health; what doctors can and cannot do for clients; how some infectious diseases are influenced by psychological factors; how clients can treat themselves as a whole person and get their doctors to do the same; why physician- and hospital-caused illness is on the increase; why laboratory tests can be "fishing trips" when unsupported by a medical history; why giving up can lead to serious illness and death; how pain can be managed by changes in attitude, rather than with medication alone.

The Physical Assessment: A Programmed Unit of Study for Nurses by Marie H. Seedor (New York: Teacher's College Press, 1974). Although this book is meant to be used by nurses, there is no reason why it cannot be adapted for use by others. It has excellent photographs that show exactly what to look for in physical assessment. Also, since it is programed, clients move through the learning process at their own pace and do not require an instructor.

Quick Work-Break, Relax/Recharge and General Meditative Relaxation; Question/Answer Adviser. Tapes developed by Win Wenger to enhance relaxation and produce other wellness effects. Available from Psychegenics Institute, Box 332, Gaithersburg, Md. 20760.

The Teenage Body Book by Kathy McCoy and Charles Wibbelsman, M.D. (New York: Pocket/Wallaby, 1979). Gives straightforward and comprehensive information on sex, parents, shyness, suicidal feelings, venereal disease, ear-piercing, excess hair, masturbation, plastic surgery for nose or breasts, weight, perspiration, and contraceptives. Suggested age range is 12 to 21.

The Well Body Book by Mike Samuels, M.D., and Hal Bennett (New York: Random House, 1973). Presents a great deal of practical information and is especially useful in showing how to *do* and understand what a doctor or nurse practitioner does when completing a physical exam; how to diagnose and treat minor symptoms and emergencies; when to see a doctor; and, how the body works—for example, what blood does, how lymph works, how antibodies work, what happens when you cut yourself, excellent drawings of the male and female anatomy, and how the endocrine system works.

The Wellness Newsletter published by The Wellness Institute. Provides information on ways to enhance wellness, recent research in the area, upcoming workshops and other topics of interest. Available from Dr. Carolyn Chambers Clark, The Wellness Institute, Cranberry Lake, P.O. Box 132, Sloatsburg, N.Y. 10974.

SELF-HELP GROUPS

COPE (Coping with the Overall Pregnancy/Parenting Experience). Founded by a psychiatric nurse who felt isolated and bewildered during her first pregnancy. The organization now sponsors a variety of services for parents, including a hot line for emergencies; counseling services; programs run in collaboration with local clinics and high schools for young, single, pregnant women; mothers-of-toddlers' groups; fathers' groups; postabortion counseling, and more. Write: 37 Clarendon St., Boston, Mass. 02116.

FA (Families Anonymous). A self-help group for parents whose teenagers have been in fairly serious and repeated trouble related to drug use, destructive behavior, or criminal offenses. Write: Box 344, Torrance, Calif. 90501 or call: 213-775-3211.

C-SEC (Caeserean Section, Education, Concern). Formed by parents who had Caeserean deliveries. Aim is to make delivery as pleasant and meaningful as possible. Write: 15 Maynard Rd., Dedham, Mass. 02026.

Handicapped Children's Early Education Program. Parents can contact this organization to find an advocate in their state who will help them unravel the red tape necessary to obtain services for their handicapped child. Contact the program at: 400 Maryland Ave., S. W., Washington, D.C. 20202.

Health-Pac. Provides research and analyses of American Health System for Women's groups and other consumers for use in forming their own self-help groups. Write: Health-Pac, 17 Murray St., New York, N.Y. 10017 or 558 Capp St., San Francisco, Calif. 94110.

LLL (La Leche League). Begun by nursing mothers to help parents with breast-feeding. Staffed by women who have successfully nursed their babies. Look in your phone book or write: La Leche League International, 9616 Minneapolis Ave., Franklin Park, Ill. 60131 or call: 312-455-7730.

National Runaway Hotline. Funded by HEW, provides advisory

services to runaways and parents on a 24-hour, confidential, free basis. Call: 800-621-4000 (U.S.) or 800-972-6004 (Illinois).

Overeaters Anonymous. Patterned after AA. Groups meet regularly to offer mutual support in diet plan. Write: Overeaters Anonymous, 2190 190th St., Torrance, Calif. 90504 or call: 213-320-7941.

National Self-Help Institute. Developed to provide group leadership and administrative training programs for self-help groups, provide research findings, work to develop a supportive relationship between professionals and self-help organizations, and publish a national inventory of self-help groups. Write: Leonard Borman Research Associate Center for Urban Affairs, Northwestern University, 1040 Sheridan Road, Evanston, Ill. 60201.

P.A.C.T. (Parents and Children Together). An association for support, help, encouragement of parents of children with congenital heart defects. Write: 25 Coolidge Road, Arlington, Mass. 02174 or call: 617-646-4186.

PA (Parents Anonymous) provides help for parents who abuse their children or are afraid of doing so. Toll-free number: 800-421-0353.

Parents without Partners is a national movement to help the single parent. Each local chapter provides its members with regularly scheduled speakers, panelists, or films to help the single parent understand and cope with the situation of being a single parent. Recreation, social, and family activities are also planned. Other services offered by some communities are assistance with dealing with divorce and a preventive effort in schools to help young people contemplate marriage in a serious, nonromantic, nonmythical way. For more information, write: Parents without Partners, Inc., 7910 Woodmont Ave., Washington, D.C. 20014. 301-654-8850.

Self-Help Reporter A guide to groups developed to provide help for themselves. Write: Self-Help Reporter, National Self-Help Clearing House, Graduate School and University Center/CUNY, 33 W. 42nd St., Rm. 1227, New York, N.Y. 10036.

United Ostomy Association, Inc. Assists in the rehabilitation of those who have had ileostomy, colostomy, or urinary ostomy surgery through mutual aid, moral support, and education about ostomy surgery, its care and management. 424 local chapters in the U.S. and Canada. Write: United Ostomy Association, Inc., 1111 Wilshire Blvd., Los Angeles, Calif. 90017 or call: 213-481-2811.

V.D. Hotline funded by HEW. Provides confidential, anonymous, free consultation, information, and referral services on all aspects of sexually transmitted diseases. Call: 800-523-1885 (U.S.) or 800-462-4966 (Pennsylvania).

Widow-to-Widow, offers help and information to widowed persons and provides them with the opportunity to learn from others in similar situations. Write: Widow-to-Widow, Widowed Resources Center, 25 Huntington Ave., Boston, Mass. 02115 or call: Dr. Phyllis Silverman, American Institutes of Research, 617-661-6180.

SEXUALITY

Atlas of the Ovulation Method by Evelyn and John Billings (Collegeville, Wisc.: The Liturgical Press, 1974). These two Australian doctors have developed the ovulation method of birth control that helps women to become familiar with variations in their cervical mucus and to use the quality of their mucus to determine whether it is a safe or unsafe day for unprotected intercourse.

Liberating Masturbation: A Meditation on Self Love by Betty Dodson (New York: Bodysex Designs, 1974). Offers encouragement and suggestions for masturbation. This book is available from Bodysex Designs, P.O. Box 1933, New York, N.Y. 10001 for $4.00.

My Secret Garden: Women's Sexual Fantasies by Nancy Friday (New York: Pocket Books, 1974). A book that can be read before or during a sexual experience.

Sex Therapy at Home by David J. Kass and Fred Strauss (New York: Simon and Schuster, 1975). A clinically tested program that shows clients a self-directed way to sexual enjoyment. No sex therapist or professional helper is needed. Clients are given the tools to take their own and their partner's sexual profile. Clients are guided step by step through a sexual enhancement program.

Sexuality and the Spinal Cord Injured Woman by Sue Bregman (Minneapolis, Minn.: Sister Kenny Inst., 1975). This 24-page pamphlet is designed for physically disabled women and health professionals who work with them. The author deals with many issues in a down-to-earth, direct, and practical way; suggestions are based on information she gathered from interviewing women who had spinal cord injuries. Topics covered include: setting the mood, methods of sexual stimulation, orgasm, managing physical problems without stifling romance, and social techniques. Available from the Sister Kenny Institute, Dept. 199, 1800 Chicago Avenue, Minneapolis, Minn. 55404.

Total Orgasm by Jack Lee Rosenberg (New York: Random House, 1973). This book discusses why people have trouble enjoying sex. Exercises are provided for readers (and their partners) to use to enhance sexual pleasure.

WELLNESS/HEALTH ASSESSMENT

Health Hazard Appraisal, developed by Drs. Lewis Robbins and Jack Hall. Questions in the Appraisal probe life style information and this is used to compile your present risks and show implications of continuing these behaviors. For more information, see: J. DaLou, J. N. Sherwood, and L. Hughes, "Health hazard appraisal in patient counseling." *Western Journal of Medicine*, 1975, vol. 122 (February): 177–180.

Life Change Index, developed by Dr. Thomas H. Holmes, University of Washington School of Medicine, Seattle, Washington. The Index has been published in several places including the *Chicago Tribune*, April 27, 1976, and *High Level Wellness* by Donald B. Ardell, published in 1977 by Rodale Press, Emmaus, Pa. The Index rates 43 life changes and predicts a person's risk of becoming ill.

Voice Stress Analysis, developed by Introspective Technology Services, 2172 Green St., San Francisco, Calif. 94123. A voice analyzer measures minute changes in voice patterns, pinpointing stress patterns and attitudes. Exercises are tailored to each person's need to deal with emotions and attitudes that may be producing stress.

Wellness Inventory, developed by The Wellness Resource Center, 42 Miller Avenue, Mill Valley, Calif. 94941. A 100-page workbook containing all the questionnaires used at the center as well as specific guidelines for how to increase one's wellness.

YOGA, MASSAGE, HEALING

The Massage Book by George Downing (New York: Random House, 1972). The complete book of massage—materials, strokes, reducing body tension, using music, self-massage, massage for animals and lovers, anatomy, meditation, and other forms of massage.

Our Earth, Our Cure by Raymond Dextreit (Brooklyn, N.Y.: Swan House Publishing, 1974). A guide to the vegetarian way of life compiled from the works of a European naturopath. It is focused on finding cures in nature, taking the stand that enduring cures are only possible when people are in accord with nature. This book presents some relatively radical ideas, especially regarding the use of clay for curative purposes. Available from the publisher, P.O. Box 170, Brooklyn, N.Y.

The Practical Encyclopedia of Natural Healing by Mark Bricklin (Emmaus, Pa.: Rodale Press, 1976). This encyclopedia gives information on a wide variety of subjects, including acne, athlete's foot, back pain, bedwetting, and biofeedback.

Slimming With Yoga by Dodi Shultz (New York: Dell, 1968). This is a pocket-sized introduction to yoga postures. Its advantages are its size and price and the good illustrations of postures.

Yoga for Americans by Indra Devi (Englewood Cliffs, N.J.: Prentice-

Hall, 1959). This book answers basic questions about what yoga is and provides a six-week course in hatha yoga. There are photographs of various postures and descriptions of how each can be used for body ailments. There is also an excellent discussion of diet after age 35.

Yoga, Youth, and Reincarnation, by Jess Stern (New York: Bantam, 1965). This book provides a wealth of information on the yoga way of life. It has excellent illustrations and directions of yoga postures. Suggests beginning, intermediate, and advanced poses, and discusses the potential uses of yoga postures to enhance health.

NAME INDEX

SUBJECT INDEX